CHICKEN SOUP FOR THE EXPECTANT MOTHER'S SOUL

101 Stories to Inspire and Warm the Hearts of Soon-to-Be Mothers

Jack Canfield
Mark Victor Hansen
Patty Aubery
Nancy Mitchell

Health Communications, Inc.
Deerfield Beach, Florida

www.hci-online.com
www.chickensoup.com

We would like to acknowledge the following publishers and individuals for permission to reprint the following material. (Note: The stories that were in the public domain, or that were written by Jack Canfield, Mark Victor Hansen, Patty Aubery and Nancy Mitchell are not included in this listing.)

Baby's Choice. Reprinted by permission of Colleen M. Story. ©1996 Colleen Story.

It Will Change Your Life. Excerpted from *Everyday Miracles* by Dale Hanson Bourke. ©1999 used by permission of Broadman & Holman Publishers.

I'm Ready. Reprinted by permission of Kristen Cook. ©1999 Kristen Cook.

It's a . . . Father! Reprinted by permission of *Texas Monthly.* Originally appeared in the December 1977 issue of *Texas Monthly* by Stephen Harrington.

The Journey Begins and *Love in the Rearview Mirror.* Reprinted by permission of Jim Warda. ©2000 Jim Warda.

Inner Sight. Reprinted by permission of Ami McKay. ©2000 Ami McKay.

Delayed Gratification. Reprinted by permission of Patricia K. Cameransi. ©1998 Patricia K. Cameransi.

(Continued on page 362)

Library of Congress Cataloging-in-Publication Data

Chicken soup for the expectant mother's soul: 101 stories to inspire and warm the hearts of soon-to-be mothers / [compiled by] Jack Canfield . . . [et al.].
   p.   cm.
ISBN 1-55874-797-4 (hardcover)—ISBN 1-55874-796-6 (trade paper)
   1. Mothers. 2. Pregnant women. 3. Pregnancy. 4. Childbirth. 5. Infants (Newborn)—Care. I. Canfield, Jack
HQ759.C524 2000
306.874'3—dc21

              00-039543

©2000 by Jack Canfield and Mark Victor Hansen

ISBN 1-55874-796-6 (trade paper) — ISBN 1-55874-797-4 (hardcover)

Publisher: Health Communications, Inc.
          3201 S.W. 15th Street
          Deerfield Beach, FL 33442-8190

Cover redesign by Lisa Camp
Inside book typesetting by Lawna Patterson Oldfield

With love,

We dedicate this book to all expectant mothers.

May your days of waiting for your new arrival

be filled with health and happiness,

and we wish you and your family many blessings.

Contents

8. ON MOTHERHOOD

9. EXPECTANT WISDOM

Acknowledgments

Chicken Soup for the Expectant Mother's Soul took us over three years to complete. It has been a labor of love for all of us, and without the support we received, this book could not have been created.

We would like to acknowledge all of you who continue to support us and allow us the time to create such wonderful books.

Our publisher, Peter Vegso, who continues to support us and keeps the *Chicken Soup* factory cooking.

Heather McNamara, our dear, dear friend who spent countless hours editing, reading and searching for better stories to make this book what it is. We love you, Heather, for all of your hard work and support. You kept the faith, and we couldn't have done this without you.

To D'ette Corona, Heather's assistant, for all of your typing, reading, searching for stories, and most of all, for your support when we needed it most.

To Sondra Keeler, who read hundreds of stories, for your typing and for always being there when we needed you.

To Chrissy Donnelly, our friend and our colleague, who contributed many stories to this book and was a major supporter on this project.

To Christine Belleris, Allison Janse, Lisa Drucker and Susan Tobias, our editors at Health Communications, Inc., for working so closely with Heather and D'ette to make this book the best it could be. We appreciate you so much.

Sharon Linnéa, our outside editor, who continually supports us with feedback and quality stories. Thank you, Sharon. You are the best!

Leslie Forbes Riskin, who supports us to no end. Leslie, you are wonderful and we are truly grateful to you for your support.

Veronica Romero and Joanie Andersen, for continuously taking care of Patty Aubery and the day-to-day operations, book tours and scheduling, so we could stay focused on writing and editing.

Teresa Esparza, Robin Yerian, Deborah Hatchell, Cindy Holland and Michelle Kiser, who tended to all of the operational duties that had to be handled daily throughout the entire project. You guys are truly amazing!

Patty Hansen, the president of our legal and licensing department, who manages the business side of our world so we can focus our time on completing such wonderful books.

Lisa Williams, Michelle Adams, and Christi Joy for taking good care of Mark, which allows him to travel the world to spread the word of *Chicken Soup for the Soul.*

Laurie Hartman, for overseeing our licensing department and taking good care of our *Chicken Soup* brand.

To all of our coauthors: Thank you for continuing to support us and for sending stories our way that were better suited to *Chicken Soup for the Expectant Mother's Soul.*

To the marketing, sales and PR staff, especially Kim Weiss, Terry Burke, Larry Getlen and Randee Feldman, who continue to spread the word about the *Chicken Soup* series.

To our initial readers—Linda Mitchell, Barbara LoMonaco, Kelly Zimmerman, D'ette Corona, Chrissy Donnelly and

Sondra Keeler—for reading through thousands of stories to help us find the perfect stories to create the best book possible, and who offered moral support whenever we needed it.

To all of the contributors who have allowed us to include their stories as part of our book.

A special thanks to Carol Kline for the wonderful introduction to the book and your ongoing support of the project.

To all of the people who dedicated a few weeks of their busy lives to reading, evaluating and commenting upon the final selection of stories. Your feedback was priceless. Barbara Astrowsky, Ruth Beach, Christine Belleris, Karla Bleecker, Rudy and Alice Borja, Alyson Bostwick, Denise Boyd, Gina Brusse, Diana Chapman, D'ette Corona, Ray and Alma Dagarag, Kira Fay, Kelly Garman, Rhonda Glenn, Tina Gorbet, Connie Heskett, Bevin Huston, Allison Janse, Donna Johnson, Karen Johnson, Sondra Keeler, Camie Worsham-Kelly, Sharon Landeen, Fran Little, Sharon Linnéa, Barbara LoMonaco, Patricia Lorenz, Michelle Martin, Heather McNamara, Linda Mitchell, Jeanne Neale, Penny Porter, Martica Reardon, Dee Riskin, Andrea Spears, Maureen Wilcinski and Kelly Zimmerman.

Thank you to our fellow publishers for their continued support in the permissions process—Anthony Pekarik at Simon & Schuster, Faith Barbato at HarperCollins, Patricia Flynn and Carol Christiansen at Random House. Reagan Marshall and Mary Suqqett of Universal Press and Taryn Phillips Quinn at *Woman's World* magazine. Thank you.

To all of the people we haven't mentioned but without whom we could not have completed this project, including all of the wonderful writers who submitted their work to be included in the book, and everyone at Health Communications, Inc. We are grateful for the many hands that made this book possible. Thank you all!

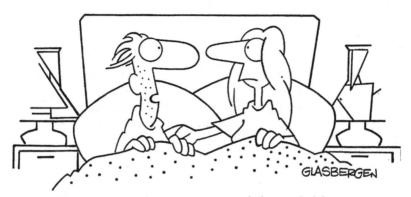

"Let's try getting up every night at 2:00 A.M.
to feed the cat. If we enjoy doing that, then
we can talk about having a baby."

Introduction

"You're pregnant." These words can be the most exciting—and perhaps terrifying—words in a woman's life. So begins the time of waiting, watching and preparing. Nothing will ever be the same again. Our bodies undergo vast changes, while our emotions run the gamut from anticipation to awe when we feel the first flutterings of life inside us, to anxiety about labor and our ability to parent. From nausea to euphoria, pregnancy is definitely a thrilling ride.

Whether you're pregnant or awaiting adoption, *Chicken Soup for the Expectant Mother's Soul* will be a steadfast companion for the expectant woman and, indeed, the entire family—including the parents-to-be, grandparents-to-be, as well as any siblings of the new baby who are bursting with unbridled enthusiasm to greet the newest addition. These stories will entertain, comfort and inspire you while you wait for the arrival of your precious newborn.

Most likely, if you're pregnant, you work either in or out of the home, and have a million and one things to distract you from the miracle occurring right inside your own body. Reading this book will help expectant mothers savor all the different facets of the unique experience of pregnancy.

In older cultures, women sat together to share stories of

their life experiences. The younger women benefited from the company of older and wiser women, who helped them understand the mysterious events surrounding pregnancy and childbirth. Think of this book as your own portable support group of women.

For the first-time mom, these stories will provide invaluable insights about getting pregnant, breaking the wonderful news to her spouse and family, and going through those important nine months—the unique joys, sensations and discomforts that bind all pregnant women together. In this book, women—and men—share their experiences of labor and birth, as well as dealing with a newborn.

Experienced moms will laugh and cry at these stories, reassured that they are not alone, as they relive some of their own experiences related in these pages.

Of course, dads are an important part of this journey too, so we've included stories from the father's point of view which both new and experienced dads will enjoy.

We also included some stories about complicated pregnancies, so that women facing these same kinds of challenges would find comfort in the knowledge that difficult pregnancies can still produce happy, healthy babies.

As you can see, *Chicken Soup for the Expectant Mother's Soul* has something in it for everyone, but most importantly for the expecting mom expanding emotionally and physically with the growing life inside of her. Reading these stories will validate her vision that becoming a mother brings deep and abiding rewards. It is our sincere wish that this book will help you remain inspired, excited and courageous until that indescribable moment when you can finally hold your new baby in your arms. May you have a happy and healthy pregnancy.

Jack Canfield, Mark Victor Hansen, Patty Aubery
and Nancy Mitchell with Carol Kline
Coauthor, Chicken Soup for the Mother's Soul II

Share with Us

We would love to hear your reactions to the stories in this book. Please let us know what your favorite stories were and how they affected you.

Also, please send us stories you would like to see published in future editions of *Chicken Soup for the Expectant Mother's Soul*. You can send us stories you have written or ones you have read and liked.

Send your stories to:

Chicken Soup for the *Expectant Mother's Soul*
P.O. Box 30880-EM
Santa Barbara, CA 93130
To e-mail or visit our Web site:
www.chickensoup.com

We hope you enjoy reading this book as much as we enjoyed compiling, writing and editing it.

Baby's Choice

Did you ever think, dear Mother,
As the seeds of me you sowed,
As you breathed new life inside of me
And slowly watched me grow,
In all your dreams about me
When you planned me out so well,
When you couldn't wait to have me there
Inside your heart to dwell,
Did you ever think that maybe
I was planning for you, too,
And choosing for my very own
A mother just like you?
A mother who smelled sweet and who
Had hands so creamy white,
A tender, loving creature
Who would soothe me in the night?
Did you ever think in all those days
While you were coming due,
That as you planned a life for me
I sought a life with you?
And now as I lay in your arms,
I wonder if you knew
While you were busy making me,
I was choosing you!

Colleen M. Story

1

WE'RE PREGNANT

Babies are such a nice way to start people.

Don Herold

It Will Change Your Life

Time is running out for my friend. We were sitting at lunch when she casually mentions that she and her husband are thinking of "starting a family." What she means is that her biological clock has begun its countdown, and she is being forced to consider the prospect of motherhood.

"We're taking a survey," she says, half-joking. "Do you think I should have a baby?"

"It will change your life." I say carefully, keeping my tone neutral.

"I know," she says. "No more sleeping in on Saturdays, no more spontaneous vacations."

But that is not what I mean at all. I look at my friend, trying to decide what to tell her.

I want her to know what she will never learn in childbirth classes. I want to tell her that the physical wounds of childbearing heal, but that becoming a mother will leave her with an emotional wound so raw that she will be forever vulnerable.

I consider warning her that she will never read a newspaper again without asking, "What if that had been my child?" That every plane crash, every fire will haunt her. That when she sees pictures of starving children she will wonder if anything could be worse than watching your child die.

I look at her carefully manicured nails and stylish suit and think that no matter how sophisticated she is, becoming a mother will reduce her to the primitive level of a bear protecting her cub. That an urgent call of "Mom!" will cause her to drop a soufflé or her best crystal without a moment's hesitation.

I feel I should warn her that no matter how many years she has invested in her career, she will be professionally derailed by motherhood. She might arrange for child care, but one day she will be going into an important meeting and she will think about her baby's sweet smell. She will have to use every ounce of discipline to keep from running home, just to make sure her child is all right.

I want my friend to know that everyday decisions will no longer be routine. That a five-year-old boy's desire to go to the men's room rather than the women's at McDonald's will become a major dilemma. That right there, in the midst of clattering trays and screaming children, issues of independence and gender identity will be weighed against the prospect that a child molester may be lurking in the restroom. However decisive she may be at the office, she will second-guess herself constantly as a mother.

Looking at my attractive friend, I want to assure her that eventually she will shed the pounds of pregnancy, but she will never feel the same about herself. That her life, now so important, will be of less value to her once she has a child. That she would give it up in a moment to save her offspring, but will also begin to hope for more years—not to accomplish her own dreams, but to watch her children accomplish theirs. I want her to know that a cesarean scar or shiny stretch marks will become badges of honor.

My friend's relationship with her husband will change, but not in the ways she thinks. I wish she could understand how much more you can love a man who is always careful to powder that baby or who never hesitates to play with his son or daughter. I think she should know that she will fall in love with her husband again for reasons she would now find very unromantic.

I wish my friend could sense the bond she will feel with women throughout history who have tried desperately to stop war and prejudice and drunk driving. I hope she will understand why I can think rationally about most issues, but become temporarily insane when I discuss the threats of nuclear war to my children's future.

I want to describe to my friend the exhilaration of seeing your child learn to hit a baseball. I want to capture for her the belly laugh of a baby who is touching the soft fur of a dog for the first time. I want her to taste the joy that is so real it hurts.

My friend's quizzical look makes me realize that tears have formed in my eyes. "You'll never regret it," I say finally. Then I reach across the table, squeeze my friend's hand, and offer a prayer for her and me and all of the mere mortal women who stumble their way into the holiest of callings.

Dale Hanson Bourke

I'm Ready

I stared at the stick in disbelief. Two straight, pink lines. No doubt about it—pregnant.

Oh my God!

A mix of excitement and sheer terror washed over me. Sure, my husband and I had talked about having a baby. I just didn't think it would happen so fast. It seemed like one minute we were talking and the next, I was standing in front of the drugstore's home pregnancy section debating whether I should buy the single- or the two-test pack.

I had a feeling—early mother's intuition maybe?—and bought just a single test. That was all I needed. We were having a baby. And I'd never even changed a diaper.

What were we thinking?

My husband, Joe, developed the baby pangs a year ago. I, on the other hand, was seized by fear. I wasn't ready. I'd look at a baby and mentally count the bottles of Pepto-Bismol the parents would consume once that bundle of joy hit those turbulent teens, or I'd calculate how much four years of college would cost. Then the baby bug bit me—and not a second too soon.

Now my body's on this wild, hormonal ride, and I have to say, sometimes I want to get off.

I'm close to thirty years old, but my complexion is sixteen. Nausea is my constant companion. My friends even ask for upchuck updates. I never drive anywhere without an air-sickness bag by my side, and I've thrown up in so many restaurant parking lots that I've thought about asking if I could just rent my dinners instead of buying them. My bladder has shrunk to the size of a lima bean, requiring me to pee exactly every thirteen minutes.

And I'm so acutely tuned in to pain—yeah, that bodes well for an easy labor and delivery—that I swear, early on, I could feel each and every cell dividing. Hypochondriacs are not good pregnant women.

More proof. When two barf-free weeks passed, I panicked. I felt so normal I figured something had to be wrong. Maybe I wasn't having a baby after all. Maybe it was a hysterical pregnancy. My husband assured me the only thing hysterical about this pregnancy is me.

And my maternity underwear.

I'm not sure which is scarier—having my body feel so out of control or those enormous, one-size-fits-all panties. At four months, my belly's still at that awkward is-she-pregnant-or-is-that-a-beer-gut stage. My little Buddha belly is enough to keep me out of my stylish silk undies, but it's still too small for the maternity briefs. I can pull those things up over my chest.

I think I just invented combination bra and underwear. I'll call it the brunder. If I can sell that idea to Victoria's Secret, no more worries about our kiddo' s college tuition. But I have to say, the most amazing transformation of all—even more than filling out that maternity underwear some day—is how neurotic I've become about this little person who isn't even born yet. It all hit when I saw the first sonogram of our baby on the monitor. That's when I really and truly realized this was our baby. Our baby. The nausea and frequent urination, all the inconveniences, well, they just melted away. They didn't matter anymore as I looked at this amazing person. Our baby.

At just eleven weeks old, our little miracle was already so perfectly formed, yet so small—just four centimeters—that Joe nicknamed the baby "Speck."

It was much too early to tell the gender, but I saw a little girl taking her first steps, walking to school, getting her driver's license, going to college, getting married, having babies of her own. Her whole life flashed before my eyes right on that screen. I thought about what a big, ugly world is waiting out there for Speck. One filled with cancer and war and junior high dances. How could I possibly protect her from all the bad, while letting her experience all the good?

Yes, in that instant I realized there are much scarier things than that shapeless maternity underwear. But you know what else I realized? I'm ready.

Kristen Cook

It's a . . . Father!

When we found out we were pregnant, I went to the library and looked up "embryo" in the encyclopedia. There they were, the same old charts and acetate overlays of life in the womb. I was twenty-eight and had always regarded such pictures with the casual indifference of someone scanning the map of a country he never plans to visit. But now one of these embryos was harbored in my wife's body.

It would be very small now, I thought, *smaller than a cocktail shrimp, almost an abstraction.* Yet whatever rational distance I may have felt before suddenly dissipated. I was not a father-to-be but a father-in-fact, parent of an organism that was now going about the process of assembling itself with an industriousness that was, for me, almost unbearably poignant.

That I was a father in any sense seemed an improbable thing. I did not feel old enough to have children; I had barely gotten used to being an adult. Long ago I had made a vow to myself that I would never grow up, and I looked back on that covenant now with nostalgia, half-believing I could still abide by its terms.

Deep in Sue Ellen's body, the embryo nurtured its wild runaway substance in secret. It was a thing we could not see that was rooted to us, and would change our lives forever, once it ripened into an infant and came forth. The concept was so enormous it struck us only at certain moments, and even then we could not assimilate it.

By the eighth month it was time for us to gather up our blanket and two pillows and attend the first class of the workshop that would teach us the Lamaze method of prepared childbirth. The purpose of Lamaze is to enable women to have their babies with a maximum of awareness and to relieve discomfort, by using a minimum of drugs. It sounded reasonable, enlightened and certainly the thing to do. But after the first session we were a little disillusioned—perhaps because our condition no longer seemed unique.

We were shown a movie, the standard scenario: the woman panting like a dog, the husband—the "coach"— saying, "Push, honey, push," the doctor announcing, "I can see its head," the baby coming in a great fluid rush. Everyone in the audience was in tears when the lights went up. We all sniffled and smiled wanly, as if we were members of an encounter group in the afterglow of a collective primal scream.

The sessions were explicit on the importance of the husband's role—we were indispensable for morale, for timing and monitoring, but I felt this was little more than a courtesy, a way to keep us from feeling irrelevant. Most of us realized that our wives were going somewhere without us. Childbirth was a crucible we could not follow them into. We skirted around its edges and watched our women— sullen, inspired, elated—being drawn into its center.

While the women lay on their backs on their pillows practicing the controlled breathing that was to help distract their attention from any discomforts of childbirth, we would slowly press down on their legs just above the knee to simulate a contraction. "Pant, blow," the instructor said. And my wife looked up at the ceiling, panting, blowing, soaring somewhere far above the pain I was so earnestly inflicting upon her.

When the exercise was over, I looked across the room at a dozen pregnant women lying belly up, their men attending them like witless, devoted beasts, a little in awe of their own daring—and fundamentally ignorant, despite the lectures and films, of the adventure they were going to undertake. In two months, we would all be following our wives about with collapsible bassinets and dirty-diaper bags stinking of ammonia. *It better be worth it*, I thought.

I found myself envying Sue Ellen's pain, though it was something I could not have told her. Every night we trained together, like athletes. But she alone would be on the field feeling the athlete's sweet, high-principled agony at the finish of the race. I would be there cheering, holding out the Gatorade.

It happened three weeks early, two days before our last Lamaze class. At 4:30 one morning I felt a soft, pawing motion at my shoulder and rose up out of sleep to find Sue Ellen staring at me, a worried, resolute expression on her face.

"Do your breathing," I said, very coach-like, when the first contraction struck. I got out my notebook and tried to time the pains. They were regular. I called the obstetrician, who confirmed, with drowsy competence, that a baby was about to be born. I wanted somebody to tell me it was false labor. Another two weeks or so, I thought, and I might be grown up enough to be a father.

The contractions were five minutes apart by the time we got to the hospital. Sue Ellen had wisely skipped any notice of the first eight or nine hours of labor, taking it up instead very near its peak. They hauled her up in a wheel-chair while I signed the papers in the lobby.

"They're prepping her," a nurse told me when I got to the maternity ward. "You can't go in for about twenty minutes."

For twenty minutes I just wandered around the hospital. I missed my wife intensely. My presence did not seem specious anymore. She needed me. When at last I was admitted into the labor room I saw that things were happening very quickly. Sue Ellen was lying on her side, panting. I taped a picture of a hippopotamus to the wall. This was her "focal point," and she gazed at it dutifully, her eyes still wide with distress.

The doctor came to the door as cheerful and composed as if he were the milkman. "Looks like we're going to have a baby this morning," he said. Sue Ellen took her eyes off the hippopotamus long enough to give him a dirty look. Her pain repelled all our ministrations—it had its own power that none of us could touch.

Soon I was standing in the delivery room in a green suit, holding up her shoulders while she bore down and began to push the baby out.

"Breathe, breathe," I said from behind the surgical mask, just like the fretful husband in the movie we had seen. "That's it."

"How... how long?" she asked from some far outpost of consciousness.

"Oh," the obstetrician said cheerfully, "not too long. Another few good pushes like that, and it'll be all over." He looked around the room and swiveled his stool back and forth. I was afraid he was going to start whistling.

"Now, I could give you an epidural, and it'd be over right away."

"No," she said. "I can do it."

Fifteen minutes later, looking in the big mirror at the

other end of the room, we saw the baby's head emerge.

"Push, push," we all said. I was drenched with sweat.

Suddenly our daughter was there, wailing on her mother's stomach, clay-colored, streaked with the remains of her ruined home. I watched her. She was a refugee now. In the womb she had been a perfect citizen, with all the cognizance she needed. Now she was in our care, utterly dependent on the human reflexes of devotion. They took her footprints. Her mother looked at her in a way I had never seen her look before. They handed her to me, and I held her against the sweat-stained surgical gown.

"Does she have a name?" the doctor asked.

"Marjorie Rose," I said.

That afternoon while Sue Ellen slept I went home—experiencing exaltation—to change my clothes and walk the dog. The sense of dislocation on coming back to the house was keen. I glanced at a full-length mirror and noticed that the clothes I had worn to the birth of my daughter—blue jeans, tennis shoes, a striped T-shirt—were the same kind of clothes I had worn when I was seven years old and made that vow I would never grow up. Now here I was. I took a shower and rummaged in the closet for my good pair of corduroy pants.

May 16 in Austin, Texas, was overcast, oppressively humid. I noticed this for her sake. And everything else I saw, the bare concrete parking garages, the revived gingerbread houses, the grove of live oaks in the park where the dog was now running, chasing the same squirrel she had been after for a year. I saw all of this through the baby's eyes as well as mine, as if I had never grown up and ceased noticing these things.

The dog chased the squirrel up a tree, then ran back to me. We walked through the park together, two full-grown, natural beings. I thought of one of the terms in the Lamaze glossary—"effacement." Something had been effaced in me—those clothes I had just thrown off could as well have been old skin. I was a man now, a father. In a few days, the insurance people would begin calling, "Steve, hear ya had a baby—congratulations!" and we would be getting samples of baby soap in the mail. But for now the world was dead calm, everything waiting. I drove back to the hospital to rejoin my family.

Stephen Harrigan

The Journey Begins

Most people return from Las Vegas with winnings or souvenirs. My wife came back with a baby.

After loading Gina's suitcases into our van at the airport, my wife handed me a small package. Thinking it would be a wonderfully tacky souvenir, I ripped through the paper only to find myself face-to-face with a positive pregnancy test.

Now, my wife and I had been trying to have another baby for quite some time. So, when I saw the test, my first thought was "What the heck is this?" Not very poetic, unfortunately, but very much the truth. So, I immediately looked up to find my wife smiling.

"But how?" I mumbled, knowing exactly how but not when or where.

"I was sicker than you'll ever know in Vegas," Gina whispered, so as not to let on to our boys in the backseat. "So, my mom took me to a doctor. And, with all the other tests, they wanted to make sure I wasn't pregnant. But, I guess I am."

Another baby. A third boy? A first girl? A swarm of thoughts and feelings went through my skull and down into my arteries. I'm happy. And scared. And worried that

I won't be a good enough dad. And proud of "big brother" Jeremy. And nervous that Gina and I will now be out-numbered. And sad for Matthew that he'll no longer be the baby. And hoping we'll be able to make them all feel special. And, most of all, so in awe of my wife who, once again, will show how a woman is a miracle, how she brings forth life and beauty and peace into a world so dearly in need of all three.

There aren't many things to top hearing that there's a baby on the way.

The journey begins . . . again.

Jim Warda

Inner Sight

Sometimes the greatest "inner sight" comes from the insight you gain while trying to help others. I was reading through the posts of a women's Internet group and stumbled upon a kindred spirit. There was a question posed by a young mother that caught my attention and inspired me to sit down and compose a letter of my own. She stated very simply: "I'm a thirty-something mother of two children. For months my husband and I have been considering having a third child. I am very hesitant about having another child for dozens of reasons (some being money, and mostly other selfish things). I would like to know if any moms out there are going through a similar situation of uncertainty?"

Suddenly I felt I was no longer alone in my ocean of confusion and choice. Here was someone I could relate to! Maybe it wasn't unnatural for me to be thinking so hard about having another child. I sat down at my computer and began to let the words and feelings flow.

> *Dear Stacy and Others,*
>
> *I'm contemplating motherhood. Again. Everyone in the household seems eager and willing to welcome a*

new member to our family. My son is clamoring for a little brother or sister. My husband grins from ear to ear with every glance drool-faced babies lend him as he stands in line at the supermarket. Those little cooing bundles of "cute" instinctively single him out of a crowd and put on the charm. He puts his arms around my waist and tickles my ear with a half-whispered "I'm ready."

Dinner conversations often include lobbying from my six-year-old son. "Mommy, I think I should learn to knit. I could make socks and mitts and blankets. Little ones, of course." It is a serious commitment when Poke-mania has been replaced by knitting. I teasingly read off a checklist to the family. "You're sure you are ready for mood swings and cravings and crying and late-night feedings and crying and colic and burping and more crying?" The husband smiles, "Oh, yes." The boy chimes in with an enthusiastic "Yes!"

They seem so sure, beyond the point of affirmation. How is it that they are so positive? Suddenly all eyes are on me. I look around for someone else to ask. No one steps forward. I think to myself, "Am I ready?"

When I put the question to myself I find that I am at a crossroads. How does a mother decide whether or not to bring another child into this world? I could ask a million women, but this is an answer that is ultimately found alone. This is a question that requires long walks, hot baths, meditation (and perhaps large quantities of chocolate).

At any given moment I can easily think of a logical list of reasons why being pregnant again might not be the best idea. Overpopulation, the trials of raising a child in today's society, money concerns, the differ-ence in years between children, and another ride on that carousel that reels past a million milestones a minute. . . . These all seem to argue against recurrent motherhood. There's standing room only in the back of my brain as these taunting thoughts of certainty line up to be heard. "Are you ready to crave tuna fish and watermelon for months on end? Do you really want to watch your body become some sort of alien creature's again?"

Of course there is also the list of delightful wonders that childbearing promises as well. These thoughts gently come to mind and wash the roughness of argument away. Memory offers me visions: the anticipation of a new life, the first wiggles within the womb, the love that is shared between parents, the graciousness my son will learn from having a sibling, and the quiet admiration that comes when someone else's grandmother spies your all-encompassing profile. I sit and remember what it's like to have a tiny hand grasp my finger and how the first bubbly baby smile made me weep with gladness.

In those silent moments of self-examination I am challenged to set logic and warm fuzzies aside and look to something else to guide my way. Such a decision cannot be made with cold practicality or mere emotion. I am more than thought. I am more than feeling.

Harriet Beecher Stowe once said: "Most mothers are instinctive philosophers." I believe this to be true. Whether it is labeled as instinct, intuition or Universal Truth, most mothers would agree that something beyond the prattle of life converses with their inner being. I try to steal as much quietude as I can these days waiting for the sacred dialogue to begin.

I think back to when I carried my son and how his spirit, somehow made known to me, seemed to have made the decision with me. (As if it were a task he had cosmically asked me to be a part of.) I always feel *compelled to honor his presence in my life by saying "when I was pregnant FOR him" rather than "when I was pregnant with him." We named him Ian, "gracious gift." Although I parent and teach Ian daily, I also feel gratitude in knowing him and in being one of the guides in his life. How very different pregnancy and parenting seem when I consider them as requested privileges.*

As the question comes again I look and listen into something beyond myself and ask. . . . Am I ready? Is it time to be called upon again? Is there someone waiting for my mothering touch?

Am I willing to carry this soul and shelter it with mine? Not just for nine months, but for our lives. Not giving mine up in the process, but becoming more of who I am because of it. When my heart can answer with a grateful "yes" and I feel the Universe whisper it back . . . I will be ready.

Blessings,
Ami

Ami McKay

P.S. I'll let you know the due date :)

Delayed Gratification

Any woman who has dealt with infertility knows the painful longing that accompanies the condition. When my husband and I decided it was time to think about having a baby, I never dreamed it would be a ten-year venture with infertility doctors, consultants and lawyers. Although I was brought up in a very loving family, I was an only child, and I always wanted several children of my own when I married.

Unfortunately, my mother had taken the fertility hormone DES (diethylstilbestrol) when she was pregnant with me, which was later linked to numerous medical problems in women, ranging form ovarian cancer to infertility. But because my mother was no longer alive, much of the medical information vital to my condition was unavailable. After my husband Ben and I had tried for nine months to conceive, I knew deep down that having a baby of our own would be a long ordeal.

The first year consisted of fertility drugs coupled with artificial insemination. We felt certain this would work and were discouraged when it failed. In vitro fertilization (IVF) was then suggested, which is a process where the woman is injected with fertility drugs to enable her body to produce an increased number of eggs. The eggs are retrieved and fertilized outside the body, then placed back in her womb. Our first try was successful, and we were ecstatic. I was very careful, feeling so lucky to finally be pregnant, but I unfortunately miscarried twins at eleven weeks.

The disappointment was unimaginable, but that same year I went through two more IVFs; one was an unsuccessful fertilization and the other time I miscarried. After so many months of hoping and praying, living by my cycle, doctor visits, blood tests, and discouraging phone calls, I knew that my mind and body needed a break.

For the next two years, both my husband and I changed jobs and settled into a life of two working professionals. If we couldn't be parents quite yet, we would be successful in our careers. After a move to Baltimore, we decided to look into treatments again, as well as the possibility of adoption. So, back to the same grind of injections, tests, doctor's appointments—but all with the same disheartening results: no baby.

In the meantime, we had some very dear friends, Kathy and Shawn, who had just had their second baby, a boy. They already had a three-year-old daughter, and Ben and I were their children's godparents. When we visited their home near Seattle to attend the new baby's christening, Kathy made it clear that she and Shawn felt satisfied with their family and didn't intend to have any more children. They offered to carry a baby for us if we got to the point where we might consider using a gestational carrier. Deeply grateful for their offer of love, we told them that we hadn't given up completely on trying ourselves, but that we would think about it.

We investigated adoption but learned that the average cost in the state of Maryland was between $18,000 and $25,000. We were shocked and again discouraged as that was out of the financial picture for us. After six more laborious and unsuccessful IVF attempts, with spirits depleted, I finally picked up the phone and made the most difficult call of my life. It was a cold, clear, January morning when I poured my heart out to my dear friend Kathy, and asked if she would still be willing to carry a baby for me. What a feeling to know there was someone in the world with enough love and sympathy in her heart to offer such a gift! I would be eternally and profoundly grateful.

With renewed hope, we began the process of having my frozen embryos sent overnight to a Seattle fertility clinic. Kathy would have to make a two-hour drive every day for two weeks for the procedure, which she did— graciously, generously sacrificing time with her family so that her friend might have a family. It was May 1997, and at the same time Kathy was trying to get pregnant with my embryos, I was also giving it "one last try" at home. I figured with both of us working at it, certainly something magical would happen.

No luck. Kathy and I were both unsuccessful, and for the four months following that sad time, Ben and I were dazed, numb, almost mournful. We had used all our options—we had now been trying for nine years and we were at the end of the road.

Our insurance was also running out. I had been covered for the very expensive IVF treatments, but the coverage would end in December that year. Because Kathy was so willing and encouraging, we opted to let her try one more time before the end of the year. So in October, our doctor was more than willing, once again, to perform the necessary procedure to retrieve, fertilize, freeze and ship my eggs to Seattle. Ben and I agreed this would be our last (the eleventh!) try at IVF. If it didn't work this time, we would somehow accept the grave reality that God didn't intend for us to have a family of our own; we would be grateful for what we had and devote our life to each other and our extended family.

But at the last minute there was a hitch with the insurance company: A regulation stated that in the case where a gestational carrier is being used, two embryos (of the normal ten to twelve retrieved) must be implanted in the real mother (a "good faith" act, of sorts) while the other embryos are given to the carrier. Although we had hoped all the frozen embryos could be sent to Seattle for Kathy's use, we, of course, complied with the policy.

While we awaited news of Kathy's IVF results, I was scheduled, as is routine in the IVF process, for a pregnancy test. The appointment fell on the day after Thanksgiving. Normally in an IVF, four to six embryos were implanted in me; this time, because it was just an insurance requirement, there were only two, and I knew my chances of becoming pregnant were slim to none. So as I set out at 5:30 A.M. that morning on the two-hour drive for my pregnancy test, I wondered why I was even bothering.

After arriving home many hours later, I answered the phone to a nurse's voice telling me—incredibly—that I was pregnant, that my blood hormone levels were fantastic, and that I should consider this a probable "keeper"—a true gift! Weeks later, when Ben and I heard the rapid little beat of our baby's heart through the doctor's stethoscope, we could hardly control our tears. We knew this baby was a gift from God—the results of ten years of persistence, prayers and great love.

My dear friend Kathy could curtail her noble efforts. Ben and I would have our baby's sweet smell and giggles on the carousel after all. The price we had paid through our prolonged trial and our tears would be small payment, indeed, for the beautiful, warm bundle of a very healthy Benjamin George Cameransi III, born August 2, 1998.

Patricia K. Cameransi

Enjoy Your Baby

The love of our neighbor in all its fullness simply means being able to say. . . . "What are you going through?"

Simmone Well

"Time to open presents!" one of the baby shower guests announced, and everyone gathered around as Caren Danielson and her sister-in-law, Jan Byrne, made themselves comfortable on the living-room couch. Jan was eight months pregnant . . . only it wasn't her baby. The baby actually belonged to Caren, who opened each gaily wrapped package with exclamations of delight.

Caren had the time of her life. "I've wanted to become a mom for so long," she told her friends. "And now, thanks to Jan, my dream is finally going to come true."

In Caren's baby book there is an entry her own mom made when she was only a girl. Asked about her goals in life, then five-year-old Caren had answered without hesitation: "I want to get married and have a baby."

Thirty years later, Caren's dream was just as vibrant. Her new husband, Eric, was also looking forward to starting a family. But then, suddenly, tragedy struck.

Caren was working out at a downtown Chicago gym one afternoon when a blinding pain exploded inside her head. "You've had a brain hemorrhage," a doctor explained. "You're lucky to be alive."

A DES baby (children whose mother's took an anti-miscarriage drug later discovered to be toxic), Caren suffered from several medical problems, including a blood-clotting disorder. Doctors could not conclusively determine that the blood problem had caused Caren's brain hemorrhage, but they warned it could happen again. Especially if she got pregnant.

"The stress of childbirth could kill you," one doctor pronounced bluntly.

"I survived a brain hemorrhage, maybe I could survive childbirth, too," Caren told Eric later that same night. "We could still try, in spite of what the doctor said."

"I married you because I love you, not because of any babies," Eric gently explained. "I couldn't bear losing you."

But Caren wanted a baby so much, she was willing to try almost anything. And then she remembered a TV movie she'd seen about surrogate motherhood. "Maybe that would work for us," Caren told Eric. "My health problems aren't genetic. You and I could make a beautiful baby together—we'd just need someone else to carry it to term for us."

Caren and Eric shared their plans with Eric's folks, who thought it was a great idea. They passed the word along, and a few weeks later, on Caren's thirty-sixth birthday, she and Eric came home after a night on the town and their answering machine was blinking.

The message was from Eric's sister, Jan. "Mom and Dad just told me you're looking for a surrogate mom, and I wanted you to know that I'd be honored to carry your baby for you," Jan's message began. "I think it would be the most incredible experience for me, and I know you and Eric would make great parents."

Caren played the message again and again. "So what do you think?" Eric asked, giving his wife a hug.

"I think," Caren managed through sobs, "that your sister must be some kind of an angel."

Jan is also a forty-five-year-old Madison, Wisconsin, divorced mother of three—Matthew, twenty-one, Beth, nineteen and Katie, fifteen. When her mom and dad told her about Eric's and Caren's wish to find a surrogate mom, something deep inside Jan had clicked. "I could do that for them," she decided after many hours of careful thought. "I always loved being pregnant, but I don't want any more children of my own."

Together, Caren and Jan researched surrogate parenting, and found a specialist in Milwaukee who could help. Jan underwent a thorough medical evaluation, and then Caren's eggs were harvested and fertilized in vitro using Eric's donated sperm.

Three days later, Caren and Eric paced the waiting room while the doctor implanted four microscopic embryos inside Jan's uterus. *Will any of them really grow into a baby?* Caren wondered, but only time would tell.

Caren refused to get her hopes up. Then one afternoon she called home and retrieved a phone message from the clinic nurse asking her to call back. Caren's heart pounded as she dialed the number.

"I wanted you to be the very first to hear the news," the nurse announced happily. "You're pregnant!"

Caren was ecstatic. "This is really going to happen," she thrilled. "I'm going to become a mom."

Caren and Eric accompanied Jan to every doctor's appointment. The women shopped together for maternity outfits, and every night Caren read baby books so she could follow her baby's growth.

"I'm so lucky that we have the possibility of having our own biological child," Caren wrote in a journal. "I feel such gratitude that we have Jan. Forty-five years old, putting her body, her health and her life at risk so we can have a baby. It's so unbelievable that somebody would do that."

Caren celebrated every new milestone—the baby's first kick, the first time she heard the fluttery fetal heartbeat. "We're going to have a son," she wrote after one sonogram. "You can see everything. He has all his pieces and parts. I'm really starting to fall in love. The nesting instinct has really kicked in. Even though I'm not pregnant I feel more maternal. I spent four hours today putting recipes in a book and making chicken soup."

And then, late in Jan's eighth month, a frantic call from Jan. "The doctor says I have gestational diabetes."

"What have I done to you?" Caren blurted, but the doctor assured Caren her sister-in-law would be okay. Her diabetes could be controlled with diet, but just to be on the safe side, they would induce labor two weeks before Caren's baby was due.

In the delivery room, Caren and Eric stood on either side of Jan, holding her hands and helping her with her breathing. *This is the most wonderful day of my life,* Caren thought as she watched her baby emerge into a brand new world.

Caren sat up all night in Jan's hospital room holding her newborn son. They named him Blake Jan, in honor of the woman who had made it all possible.

"How can I ever thank you enough for what you've done?" Caren sobbed the next day as she and Eric prepared to take their baby home.

"Enjoy your baby," came Jan's simple, heartfelt reply. All along Jan had felt that Blake was truly Caren's and Eric's—that she was merely the infant's caretaker. "All I did was help him along his way," she always insisted.

For Mother's Day, Jan received a beautiful bouquet. "To my birth mom," read the card. "You've given me the best life a baby could ever have."

Today, Caren can no longer imagine her life without Blake. She loves everything about being a mom, and she's still startled when she looks into his eyes and sees a little piece of herself looking back.

Now and then in the local market or along the city side-walks, a woman will rush up to Caren and gaze longingly into Blake's stroller. "My husband and I have been trying for so long to have a baby of our own," the woman will lament, and smiling, Caren will reply, "Let me tell you about this little guy right here and what it took to bring him into this world . . ."

Heather Black

Breaking the News

After hearing the news, I floated to the car flooded with questions, wondering how I was going to tell my husband and worrying about his reaction.

The outcome of the examination I had just completed would definitely change our lives.

When I arrived home, there was a message on the answering machine; he was working late at the office and wouldn't be home for dinner—*a reprieve*.

Now I had time to plan my announcement. It had to be perfect! After mulling over several ideas, I made my decision and picked up the phone. "What city please?" asked the sharp voice on the other end of the receiver.

"I need the number for Western Union," I nervously requested.

"One moment, please," she routinely answered.

I thanked her, then carefully dialed the number: busy signal. So, while waiting a few minutes, my thoughts wandered to my husband, working at his office in a stock brokerage firm. *Surely he'll be able to interpret my message,* I thought.

I had affectionately nicknamed him my Pizza Puff because of his unabashed love for the food. A veritable staple in his diet, he could eat it for breakfast, lunch and dinner every night, and still have it as a late-night snack. Whenever we went out for dinner, his first choice would be "a new pizza place" so he could compare the product in his quest for the ultimate pie.

I redialed the Western Union number wondering what his reaction would be when he read this telegram. *What would he do first? What would he say? Would he call me right away?*

"Western Union, how may I help you?"

I relayed the message while my heart drummed out an Indian war chant: RESEARCH COMPLETED stop. CONFIRMING NEW ISSUE stop. MINI PIZZA PUFF OFFERS LONG-TERM GROWTH stop. RELEASE DATE SET FOR MIDDLE OF JUNE stop. PREPARE NOW stop. LOVE YA, HELEN.

After supplying all the pertinent information, I asked, "How long before this telegram is delivered?"

"About an hour or two," the voice explained.

I placed the receiver back on the phone stand and stepped back, caught in a whirlwind of joy.

For the next half-hour or so, I paced the floor and watched the clock. I couldn't wait another second. I picked up the phone and called Dan. I made small talk then finally asked, "Has anyone stopped in the office to see you in the last two hours or so?"

"No. Why?" he asked quizzically.

"Oh, it's just that I know someone is supposed to come in and give you something."

"And who might this be?" he asked.

"I can't tell you. It'll spoil everything," I said.

"Helen, I don't want to cut you short, but I am in the middle of things here. Either tell me what's on your mind or we'll talk about it when I get home."

"All right, Dan, I'll tell you. I sent you a telegram."

"You what?"

"Just listen." I read him the message and waited.

The silence was deafening. "So what's that supposed to mean?"

I couldn't believe he didn't understand. "I'll read it again. Think about it!" I tried to stay calm.

"Okay, you read; I'll write it down. Maybe something will click if I see it in writing." He repeated my message. "New Issue. Mini Pizza—hey, that's my name!—June—Long-term growth, hold on Helen, there's another call coming in. Be right back."

Business, I thought, *always getting in the way of important things.*

"Okay, I'm here," came his cheerful response. "Now, let me look at this."

I waited for what seemed like forever, desperately hoping the light would dawn. Finally he commented idly, "Sounds like a new me on the way in June."

"Yes!" I shouted. "Yes! Yes! Yes!"

"You mean like a baby? Like you're going to have a baby?"

"Not exactly, I mean *we're* going to have a baby!"

"Are you sure? When did you find out? Are you okay?"

"Yes, I'm sure. Just came home from the doctor's office. And yes, I'm okay."

"Wow, Helen! This is great. Hold on."

I could hear him shouting to his coworkers, "I'm going to be a father. Helen and I are pregnant!" I could also hear the shout of congratulations.

"Helen?" he asked.

"Still here," I said.

His voiced cracked, "I'm on my way home!"

All the worries of the evening faded instantly. "Hurry home, Daddy," I whispered into the phone.

"I will, little mother," came his equally hushed reply.

Helen Colella

Great Expectations

The first thing we decided when we found out I was pregnant was to wait until the third month before we told anyone.

Ten minutes later, I was combing through my address book, calling everyone from our Realtor to my sixth-grade teacher.

"What do you mean you're worried about the change in your lifestyle?" several friends with kids said smugly. "What makes you think you'll have a life?"

I knew they were wrong. I'd be different; I am organized. I read all the books.

"Being pregnant is the easiest part," my mother-in-law said cheerfully during my bouts of morning sickness.

When I could pick my head up out of the sink, I reveled in the attention of my husband. He fussed if I so much as sneezed. "Stop it," he'd say. "You're cutting off the baby's oxygen." He developed a new habit of looking down my throat and saying clever things like, "Hello in there."

Life and work continued, except that I now had an excuse not to eat sushi. One night we went to a dinner reception. No one asked what I did for a living, though several people did ask what it was my husband did. I fled to the ladies' room, where a strange woman accosted me in order to share the intimate and horrifying details of her fifty-seven hour labor, concluding with relish, "so finally I told the doctor 'Give me the knife, I'll do it myself'."

At least these people had noticed. Not like the rest of the commuting world. No one on the train wanted to make eye contact; after all, you can't offer a seat to a pregnant woman if she's invisible. One day a blind man got on the crosstown bus, and the person next to me tapped me to get up and give him my seat. Which I did. From this I concluded that men were genetically unable to give up seats. This theory was confirmed one rainy rush hour, when I hailed a cab, and a man in a pinstripe suit shoved me aside. "You wanted women's lib, now you got it," he snarled.

Urging me to relax, my considerate husband rented a movie he thought I'd like. Or he'd like. I squirmed through the entire screening of *Alien*. But I didn't say anything. After all, this was the same man who every night put aside *Barron's* to read *Goodnight Moon* out loud to my belly.

Around this time, my husband also developed the insatiable urge to buy high-priced electronic gadgets. One night he brought home a camcorder and spent forty-six minutes photographing my abdomen. Getting into the spirit of things, I brought home an ultrasound picture of the baby. "But it looks like a herring," he said. I asked the doctor for another. This time my unborn child looked like Jimmy Durante.

I read more books. The toilet-training travails of my friends became fascinating. I debated the merits of Super Pampers with the same friend with whom I used to discuss Proust. She took me out shopping to a mall, where total strangers touched my belly like some religious totem. We bought shoes; although I wore an eight, the nine was so comfortable that my friend urged me to take the ten.

I waddled into my eighth month. My doctor chose this

time to inform me that she would be taking a two-week vacation that started a week before my due date. My usually calm husband began preparing labor contingency plans that involved beepers, cellular phones and highway detours that would challenge a SWAT team.

We took Lamaze. I read more books. The coach quizzed us. I quizzed the class. "What is Bellini?" I asked. "A champagne and peach cocktail?" someone said. "No, a Russian dish served with caviar and sour cream," said another. "I have it!" said another woman. "An upscale line of baby furniture that won't deliver on time."

In my ninth month, my father decided it was the height of hilarity to ask repeatedly, "You're sure it's not twins?" On Tuesdays everyone told me I was carrying a girl. On Thursdays everyone told me I was carrying a boy. I put away the books; my attention span had been reduced to the length of the average television commercial. I learned in my Lamaze class that effleurage is not a type of floral perfume. The same night, my husband gleefully announced to the class that the first thing I planned to do after I went into labor was to shave my legs.

Ah, labor. "It's like gas," my aunt said. "Menstrual cramps," said my mother. "Nothing to it."

They lied.

I forgot how to breathe. My husband with the high-priced dual-action stopwatch fell asleep timing contractions. My doctor never came back from Paris. The backup doctor I'd never met before was three years younger than I, just starting private practice that very night. He offered Demerol. Being offered Demerol for labor is like being offered aspirin after you've just been run over by a freight train. About the time I started pushing, a medical student wandered in. "I know this isn't the best time," she said vaguely. "I have to take a medical history."

I pushed and panted. "Your pelvis is too small," said the doctor.

"With these hips?" I asked, incredulous.

The anesthesiologist prepped me for a cesarean. "As long as we're all here, how about a liposuction, too?" I asked.

Finally they handed me a swaddled lump who looked uncannily like E.T. The nurses were still counting clamps and sponges. A metal ring was missing. Pandemonium in the operating room.

"Get an x-ray plate up here. I don't want to have to open her up again," the doctor said crossly.

"Me neither," I said. "Couldn't you just roll me through the airport metal detector?"

Five days later, we brought home our son. Waiting for us were assorted grandparents, flower baskets and the hospital bill. They charged us for the x ray. (No ring was found.)

Reading prepared me for much of this . . . except how passionately I would fall in love with my child. Nor did it tell me this crucial fact: sex is like riding a bicycle. It doesn't matter how long it's been, it comes back to you.

Liane Kupferberg Carter

2

NINE MONTHS AND COUNTING

*Let us make pregnancy an occasion when
we appreciate our female bodies.*

Merete Leonhardt-Lupa

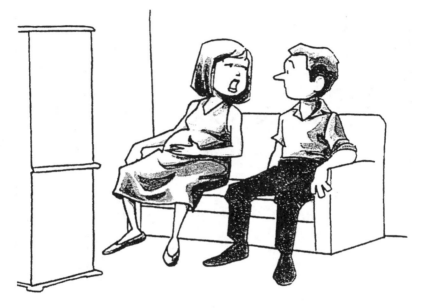

"I've gotten a whole new appreciation for the phrase 'bottom of the ninth, bases loaded.'"

Did You Just Eat a Watermelon?

I'm pregnant. Very Pregnant. And yes there are degrees of pregnancy. There's the Little Bit Pregnant where you don't show yet, you're always tired and you hang your head over the toilet. (Personally I've been fortunate enough to avoid the toilet part, and I always show, even when I'm not pregnant, to the point where people ask when the baby is due.) There's the Definitely Pregnant, where you show, supposedly you glow, you're always tired and you eat like a pig. Then there's the Let's Get Ready For Baby Pregnant, where your belly gets in the way, you're always tired, you're counting down the weeks and struggling frantically to get the nursery ready. Then there's the Very Pregnant. Not only does your belly get in the way, but it can become a lethal weapon. You're *always* tired. You don't know what day it is so you can't count anymore. You can't breathe. Your back aches.

As I said before, I'm pregnant. Very Pregnant. This is not my first. This is my seventh. Put your eyes back in your head. Yes, this is my seventh. God fooled me with the first two. Aside from being tired, I felt wonderful. I barely showed, even at full term, and I could get up and down from the floor as easily and gracefully as a ballerina could. Then number three came. He ruined pregnancy for me forever. I had water retention . . . in my ears. I, who had never waddled, started to resemble a duck. And my belly made it into a room two minutes before I did. By the way, did you realize that a full-term pregnancy is forty weeks, and if you divide that by four weeks (the average month) you end up with *ten* months. Not nine. Ten. The other pregnancy math I've never understood, is when I deliver a seven and a half pound baby and only lose five pounds in the process.

When you're pregnant, you get accustomed to hearing the same comments over and over. "When is the baby due?" My response now: "This year." "What is it?" I answer, "Well, it's either a boy, or a girl." "You're very big." (This can come in several forms. "Are you carrying twins?" "You look ready to pop," and the "You haven't had that baby *yet?*") In answer to these I find the best response is, "Yes, you're right, I'm enormous. I hadn't realized that. Thank you for pointing it out."

But the worst thing is when people I barely know touch my belly. I guess they figure that since it's out there, it's for public use. Would they touch my belly if I weren't pregnant? One of my friends commented "Maybe they're making a wish, or hoping for good luck." I think the next time people touch my belly, I'll touch theirs.

Perhaps I wouldn't find all this so disheartening if people would ask about me. But once the information about the baby is out, they walk away. It's like I no longer exist as a human being because my stomach sits in my lap.

For now I sit, waiting patiently (okay, not so patiently) for signs that my baby is ready to greet the world and reveal its gender. And for those of you who will insist on asking, "When is the baby due?" All I can say is, "Oh, this isn't a baby. I just ate a watermelon."

Anna Wight

Flying

The trick for grown-ups is to make the effort to recapture what we knew automatically as children.

Carol Lawrence

Recently, my two-year-old son and I were strolling down a sidewalk together. Both in our own little worlds, we hadn't spoken until I felt a tugging at my hand. Looking up at me, he exclaimed, "Run, Mommy, run!" Gazing back down at him, I almost had to laugh.

At six and one-half months pregnant, I can barely manage a quick walk, let alone a full-fledged run. Activities I used to take for granted, such as getting up from a chair without a grunt of effort, are things of the past. Even my family is shocked at the enormity of my belly. A friend likes to tease me about twins.

He tugs my hand more urgently and repeats, "Run, Mommy!" I start to shake my head no, but then I hesitate. How many times have I told him "no" lately?

"No, Nicholas. We can't play that rough—it could hurt the baby."

"No, I can't give you a horsey ride. You see, my back aches constantly now.

"No, Nicholas. I don't want to color—I just want to rest."

These months of pregnancy have been bittersweet. I deeply love this coming child and delight in every little nudge and kick. But it has occurred to me that this is the last time in Nicky's childhood that it will be just the two of us. Soon enough he will have to learn to share . . . Mommy's lap, Mommy's hugs, Mommy's attention.

Then I look, really look, at him. I study his outstretched hand, so pudgy and dimpled. I suddenly realize that one day it will be larger than my own. I look into his clear brown eyes, so free from our adult world of worries. They are lit up, in love with life and so excited. "Please don't ever grow up," I want to tell him. "Please always stay my little boy." He is so beautiful at this moment it actually makes my heart physically hurt.

I kneel down to his level. (Difficult, I admit, but I manage.) Then I take a moment to think at his level. We adults spend so much time worrying—about money, our careers, our responsibilities. None of this means anything to him. He is two, and he wants to run. With me, his mommy. This means something to him. And now it means something to me.

I grab his little hand tightly in my own. "Yes, Nicholas," I say. "I'll run with you." He waits for me to stand, and then we're off! His sturdy legs pound the pavement fiercely as I do my best to keep up.

It flashes through my mind that to other people we might look pretty ridiculous. A running toddler pulling his pregnant mother (who is by now huffing and puffing) along behind him. Nicholas looks at me with a huge grin. "Run, Mommy, run!" and laughs. Faster and faster we go. I am laughing out loud now, too. I forget about my aching back and my huge stomach. I forget about everything except how much I love my son. Though I lag behind, not once does he let go of my hand.

We finally do pass someone, a silver-haired lady. Instead of a strange look, she gives us a genuine smile. Maybe our joy is contagious, or maybe she remembers her own son at that age. Or maybe, just maybe, she sees what's really happening. While Nick and my feet are busy running, our hearts are busy flying.

Nicole Smith

My Baby Brother

My baby brother is not here yet,
I've seen him in pictures, but we've never met.

I've seen all his toes on both of his feet.
I cannot wait until the day we meet.

I've seen his eyes, his nose, and his mouth,
and a little something toward the south.

I've seen his arms, legs, and belly too,
just three more months until he is due.

I've seen the connections with the umbilical cord
the way he lies there—he must be bored!

I've heard the sound of his heart . . . beating fast,
I cannot wait till we meet at last.

I've even felt him move inside of my mother,
I cannot wait to meet my baby brother.

John Conklin, age thirteen

The Eleventh Hour

Dear God, I pray for patience and I want it right now!

Oren Arnold

I was nine months pregnant with my first child. My once-slim, attractive body had bloated like a blowfish. I could no longer reach my feet over my gargantuan belly. It seemed as if I had swallowed the whole Earth; my roundness was awe-inspiring. Tying my shoelaces made me look like a crazy dog chasing its tail. Around and around I'd go searching, searching, for the strings. They mocked me with their click-clack, click-clack, against the floor. My once-normal daily activities had become major undertakings. Getting out of my waterbed required skill, balance and precise timing. I would stick my legs straight up in the air and begin a rocking motion. With a-one and a-two and a-three, I'd build up enough centrifugal force to defy gravity, break the sound barrier and hurl myself off the side of the bed and onto the floor on my knees in a perfect dismount. And the stretch marks! Well, if you stood my naked body next to a globe we'd be twins. I was definitely not enjoying the last month in my third trimester.

Yet up until the ninth month, the thirty-third week, the two hundredth and twenty-second day, the eleventh hour, the . . . well you get the point. Until I got so fat I couldn't move, I loved being pregnant. I loved getting sick in the mornings. It meant my body was really hard at work making my baby. I loved the way my swollen stomach moved from side to side looking like some strange peaked mountain. The most exciting times were when I could actually feel a little elbow, the heel of a tiny foot, the roundness of a little head or bottom. I was never sure which.

However, in my ninth month, thirty-third week, two hundredth and, well, a week past my due date anyhow, I was more than tired of being pregnant. I had become convinced that this baby and I would coexist in this uncomfortable state for all eternity. My husband, Lee, and I were constantly on guard. Every hiccup, sneeze, cough, burp and gas pain had us checking our watches in the hopes that the miracle of labor had finally come. Then one night, lying on my waterbed, trying to sleep, something happened! PAIN, like I'd never experienced before.

"Owwww! Lee!" I smacked him. "Lee! WAKE UP!!!"

Out sprang Lee from the bed with a speed that rivaled a locomotive. He tripped over his pant-legs that he was trying to pull up, but undaunted he leapt forth like a runner from the gate. His eyes were unfocused and glazed as he groped around frantically for his glasses. With his hair going in every direction, his pants pulled halfway up and his eyes darting from left to right like a cornered animal, I didn't know if I could trust him to tell him what was really happening.

Sticking one leg up in the air and trying to rock back and forth, I did my best to call upon the dismounting skills I had obtained during my pregnancy. All I succeeded in doing was creating a tidal wave effect in the bed.

"Lee! Help me up here, would ya?" He seemed to have forgotten me in his frantic search for his glasses.

"Found my glasses! Keys, I need keys! And a shirt, where's my shirt?"

"Lee! Just HELP me UP would you! I'm not in labor! I just got a stupid charley horse in my leg!"

He stopped as if he'd just slammed into a brick wall. Doing a 360-degree turn, he finally made it to my side. With a-one and a-two and a-three, I was on my feet and Lee was on his knees before me, rubbing my poor tortured leg . . . which only made it worse.

"Oh, just go back to bed will you!" I said ungratefully. "I'm not having a baby tonight!"

My sensitive husband fell into bed not bothering to take off his pants or his glasses and was snoring again in two minutes flat.

I hobbled around the room walking away the pain, and I thought about how funny being nine months bloated was. Would my body ever go back to "normal"? Was I ever going to quit obsessively thinking about every second, minute, hour of each day, overly aware of each bodily function I had? What kind of mother was I going to be? Was I ever going to get to be a mother? One thing for sure, this child was already teaching me important life lessons, like being patient! Better to learn that lesson before the baby got here.

The pain receded and I rolled back into bed. I fell asleep telling myself over and over . . . it has to come out some-time . . . it has to come out sometime. I cuddled as close to my husband as my girth would allow and drifted off with visions of little pink booties, soft downy baby blankets and the smell of Johnson and Johnson baby shampoo dancing through my mind. With a contented sigh, I imagined how wonderful, how beautiful, how satisfying it would be to finally sleep on my stomach again!

Melanie L. Huber

Garbage Day

Garbage collectors were picking up our trash as my wife walked back into our house. A particular barrel was very heavy. "Lady, we can't take this," one man called out. "It's way over the weight limit."

My wife turned her eight-month-pregnant figure toward him. "It didn't seem that heavy when I carried it out," she said.

Without another word, the man emptied the barrel into the truck.

Gil Goodwin

Notes of an Expectant Father

One hour before our first childbirth class, I promised Virginia that I would be supportive, pleasant and affectionate. Furthermore, I agreed not to crack jokes, laugh at inappropriate times, bring up strange subjects, or take notes and write a story about the exciting, yet intensely personal, experience of having a first child.

"Just one minute," I said. "You know all those little things you want to buy for the B-word? This story will pay for them."

Okay, I could write the story but not reveal overly personal information. I would be kind to the other people in the class. I would pay attention to the teacher.

At our health maintenance organization, where the classes would be held for the next seven Wednesday evenings, we followed a pregnant woman into a room on the second floor. Then Virginia went to buy juice, leaving me alone in the room with three pregnant women. We sat around a big table.

"Nice weather we're having," I said.

"Yes," one replied softly. Her face reddened and she looked down at the table.

Aware that one wrong word might cause them to burst

into tears, I continued in a friendlier tone, "I'm really look-ing forward to this."

They all smiled, blushed and looked down at the table. Another pregnant woman entered the room and took a seat.

I figured that the ebb and flow of powerful hormones caused their shyness, but why were no other men here? Husbands no longer drop their wives off at the hospital and then pick them up a week later with the baby. Nowadays we stay by their sides, start to finish, a reward-ing and loving experience, and the responsible thing to do.

While I dared not ask where the husbands of these preg-nant women were, a little pillow talk seemed safe. Nobody had pillows, including us. Pillows and childbirth classes go together like Dalmatians and firehouses. Sooner or later you need pillows in class. Only I hoped it was later.

"We forgot to bring our pillows," I said. "Think we'll need them tonight?"

"You don't need pillows in breast-feeding class."

Childbirth class was held in the room next door. Pregnant women—more than I had ever seen gathered in one place, including the maternity section at the depart-ment store—waddled around the room or sat in chairs against the wall. Their husbands were by their sides, holding the pillows.

In each class private and sensitive topics were dis-cussed openly: emotional highs and lows, fears, aches, pains, things that dripped out of the body and other per-sonal matters—all of it good stuff to write about. Unfortunately, at the first class, I forgot to bring pen and paper to take notes.

Virginia and the rest of the class busily took notes when the teacher spoke. They wrote down the date we would watch a movie in class, the date we would learn how to deliver a baby if unable to make it to the hospital in time and other important dates. Why write that stuff down? Class was every Wednesday night. Just show up for class and something will happen. If it's the movie week, then we'll see a movie. If it's not, we won't.

Meanwhile, dynamite quotes and other subtle nuances of body language and facial expressions to record—never to come this way again—flew over my head.

Desperate not to miss any more information, I whispered to Virginia every time somebody made an unusual comment. "Write that down," I'd say. "Be sure to get that," or "Don't miss that!" One term to record at all cost, used by the teacher, was "Lactation Consultant."

"Get it, get it, get it," I demanded, whispering louder, leaning closer.

She whipped around like a cobra and hissed, "Shhhhhhhhhhh!"

Everyone turned and stared at me. Publicly scolded by my wife, I looked down at the floor. I knew what they were thinking: "She wears the pants."

Due dates were a common topic of conversation among the women. The date served as an introduction.

"When are you due?"

"April 20. And you?"

"March 30."

"My name is Ann."

"Nice to meet you, Ann."

The men also discussed due dates. "When is your wife due?" really meant, "Do you have to go through this whole thing before or after me?"

Weight gain was another frequently discussed topic, although the way the women discussed it evolved over the course of the class. Intoxicated by the joys of expectant motherhood, they initially overcame the taboo of making public one's weight and talked total poundage.

That is, until one woman announced that she weighed 191 pounds. Eyebrows rose. One hundred and ninety-one pounds. Nine pounds shy of 200 pounds. The next week they spoke mostly of net gain, pounds gained during pregnancy, which ranged from twenty to forty-five pounds. Forty-five pounds! After that, they limited the discussion to pounds gained over the last week.

The men discussed weight gain as well. Many of the husbands had kept pace with their wives.

"I gained three pounds last week," said one woman.

"That's nothing," added her husband. "I gained four."

During one class the women shifted uneasily in their seats and wore horrified expressions as the teacher vividly described the long drawn-out spasms of pain they would experience in labor. Of all the concerns I had about childbirth—a list too long to enumerate—the physical pain of labor, I can say bravely, was not one of them. That pain may be intense, but it's temporary, forty hours max. What will really take it out of the hide is paying for the B-word's college tuition in eighteen years.

"Embrace the pain," I advised Virginia, rolling my r's and waving my arms. "Rrrrevel in it. Never rrrrun from it. That's how swamis walk over hot coals."

Her responses to these sermons ranged from "Give me a break" to a more terse and less polite remark. Her grand-mother suggested that a man could only understand the pain of labor if he passed a kidney stone. Her husband had done so. When she saw him lying on the floor, doubled over, screaming, her first thought was, *Now he'll know what labor was like for me.*

The other couples in classes eventually grew accustomed to my note taking. Generally, when they took notes, my pen was still. And when their pens were still, I took notes.

Frequent discussions about private matters made those topics seem more ordinary and less sensitive. As commonly as the carpenter calls for a hammer or saw, we in childbirth class used the V-word, the S-word and the G-spot. I had even become desensitized to the B-word. Baby baby baby. . . I could say it ten times in a row.

The teacher predicted this would happen. The more we learned about giving birth, she said, the more relaxed and comfortable we would become with the subject. She even predicted that during labor women would not mind having strangers in the room; they would lose their shyness.

"When you're in the delivery room, you won't care if the horse cavalry rides through," she said. "Some of you will say things you never knew you were capable of saying. You'll slap your husbands and swear at them."

Good story idea, I noted. Talk to obstetricians about what they have seen and heard in the delivery room.

Three doctors addressed us for twenty minutes prior to one class. One of them, or one of the eight obstetricians who did not work at this facility, would deliver our baby. They answered questions while the class scrutinized them. Not that scrutinizing them made any difference. Whichever doctor was on duty would deliver our baby. Nevertheless, we ranked them.

The people's choice was the woman doctor who had given birth herself not too long ago. She established an instant rapport with the class, answering questions in a direct manner, explaining all the options. Choosing second place was difficult. Both Doctor X and Doctor Y earned points for humor. Soft-spoken, X had a subtle sense of humor. We smiled at his witticisms. Y, on the other hand, told jokes that elicited loud, raucous laughter—as raucous as a roomful of pregnant women and their husbands can get. When he answered questions, he shot up from his chair and bounced on his toes. Both lost points for wearing eyeglasses, which might fog up if things got too hot or steamy.

One noticeable trait of Doctor Y, which ultimately swayed our decision, was that his hands moved constantly.

He rubbed them together, drummed his fingers on the table, adjusted his eyeglasses, scratched his nose, patted his lap, folded them together and unfolded them, non-stop. It reminded me of a third baseman anxiously pounding his glove, keeping his head in the game, ready for a hot line drive. Doctor Y was ready to catch babies.

We gave second place to Doctor X.

At the last class, all the couples shared their feelings and asked their final questions. Over those past seven weeks, much camaraderie had developed. We planned to have a reunion in several months. Then everybody thanked the teacher and spoke of all they had learned.

What had I learned? Well, I had learned a lot, but I couldn't recall any of it—information overload. There were so many details to remember. If substance A drips out of the body and smells like B, don't worry. But if A smells like C, call the doctor. To get all the Latin, the female anatomy and the odors straight, a useful learning tool for husbands would be a scratch-n-sniff coloring book with a pop-up baby on the last page.

But no such learning tool exists. I can only hope that when the moment arrives, it will all come back to me. Until then, I'll review my notes.

Scott Cramer

My Hero

If I know what love is, it is because of you.

Herman Hesse

When my husband Larry pulled out of our driveway at 4:30 A.M., four to five inches of snow were already on the ground. Beautiful as the fresh powder was, illuminated by the headlights of his car, I knew we were in trouble. He had a fifteen-mile drive to the nearest station, Harpers Ferry, West Virginia, where he caught the commuter rail into Washington, D.C. It was twelve days from the scheduled cesarean delivery of our third child—there was no telling if I might go into labor before then. I was quite prone to fits of anxiety. These moments of panic were induced by seemingly every meteorologist's report within a seventy-five-mile radius of our home in rural West Virginia; we lived eight miles from the nearest town and an hour and a half from the hospital where I was to deliver our daughter. I even had nightmares about not being able to get to the hospital when it was time and having a paramedic do emergency surgery along the roadside in the middle of a snowstorm. February had never seemed so forbidding as it did now.

My husband, well aware of my fears, assured me that he would make it home from work that evening "no matter what," not wanting to leave me alone with our two small children and a baby about to make her appearance. Happily married for eight years, I trusted him with my life: I knew he was a man of the utmost integrity and loyalty and if he said he would be home, then he would be.

Hour by hour, far more quickly as the gray afternoon turned to darkness, the snow was mounting: ten inches, twenty-four inches, thirty! I tried to smile as my son and daughter, aged five and seven, peered excitedly out onto the back porch as I, almost hourly, measured how much new snow had fallen. For them, it was primarily an adventure that was happening all around them; their imaginations were filled with the endless possibilities of what they could do in the snow the next day. While they marveled at the drifts that were rapidly consuming my station wagon in front of the house, I began to panic. Larry had called me several times throughout the day to assure me that the train would be running and that he would make it home easily. Around 7 P.M., he phoned to tell me the train from the city had at long last arrived at the station. I was so relieved as visions of my husband stuck on a cold and darkened train overnight, huddling close to other Washington commuters to survive, quickly receded. Little did I know that he was about to embark on the most dangerous journey of his life.

Although his car had been snowed in at the station, he had convinced me that he was going to be able to get a ride home. I wanted to believe him, but I quietly wondered how anything would be able to move in this blizzard. As minutes became hours, I kept vigil at the family-room window, watching, waiting, and becoming more and more worried. The hours crawled by, and still I had no idea what, if anything, I could do. I prayed often, asking God to watch over my beloved wherever he was and to bring him home safely to us.

Around 2:00 A.M., as my rocking chair vigil wore on, I saw a dog out in the snow. I had last measured thirty-six inches of snow, yet the dog did not seem at all intimidated by the depths; in fact, he was prancing, almost frolicking it seemed, along what had once been our driveway through the woods. As the dog came closer, I realized with much amazement that it was actually my husband! He was pushing his way through the snow, which was most of the way up his chest. He finally got to the door, and as he gratefully embraced me, I couldn't believe my eyes—his hair, his eyebrows, his moustache, and his nose, were covered in snow and icicles. His whole body was wet and frozen, but he was okay.

Larry had walked home—fifteen miles—in over three feet of snow, in the dark of night, in the middle of a blizzard, to be with our unborn child and me. He had promised he would get home, and he had kept his word, as always. What a courageous and loyal husband I had that night! The love he knew I had for him in my heart had sustained him while God had protected him.

Our daughter, Anna Patricia, was born ten days later.

Patricia Franklin

I Know What You've Been Doing!

My sister was at her wit's end trying to stop my four-year-old nephew, Todd, from sucking his thumb. Finally, she told him if he didn't stop, his stomach would get very big and puffy.

The following Sunday in church, a very pregnant lady happened to be sitting in the same pew. Todd kept staring at her. When the service was over, he pulled at her arm and whispered, "Your stomach is big and puffy. . . I know what you've been doing!"

Becky Walker

A State of Bliss

It is only when the rigidity of advanced pregnancy sets in that you appreciate fully how useful it was to be able to bend at the waist.

Audrey Hull

They say ignorance is bliss. I believe this saying applies to a lot of things. I am totally blissful that I don't know the actual ingredients of a hot dog or how many dust mites are in my mattress. It thrills me that I have no clue when Elvis's birthday is, how many stomachs a llama has or the best way to clean a trout. There is a wonderful freedom in declaring, "I don't know and I don't care."

There are definitely things about becoming a mom I am glad I didn't know before I joined the ranks of the progeny enhanced.

I am very glad I did not know my son would weigh nine pounds eight ounces when he was born, or that he would have a big head. (When asked what kind of baby she wanted, a woman I know replied, "One with a small head.")

No one ever told me that I was going to have a big baby; for this lack of knowledge I am truly grateful.

What possible good would it have done me if the doctor had said at the end of my pregnancy, "Whoa—sign up for heavy drugs now because you'll have a heck of a time getting that one out!"

I could have guessed I'd have a big baby. Unlike some of my friends who just looked like they'd had a big dinner when they were nine months pregnant, I was a lot more bulbous in nature. I couldn't see my feet after about month seven and had to have the UPS man tie my shoes on more than one occasion.

It must have been hormonally induced insanity that forced me to buy a knit dress with horizontal stripes; anyone who reads *Vogue* faithfully or has done a little people-watching knows horizontal stripes make you appear wider. When I look back at pictures of myself, I realize I looked like a gigantic, mobile blue-and-white beach umbrella. The joke, "When God said 'Let there be light' he asked you to move," applied to me.

I've heard it said that childbirth is like trying to squeeze a St. Bernard through a cat door. In my case, it was more like a baby hippo.

I'm also glad I didn't know that I wouldn't like shopping for myself anymore. It happened time and time again. After having the baby, I'd go shopping for some nonmaternity clothes that had been manufactured sometime within the current presidential term. My body was still not recognizable as my own—my weight was redistributed in places that were pleasing (my chest) and not so pleasing (my thighs). I read somewhere that nursing mothers maintain fat on their thighs so they can continue to feed their babies should a famine occur. I could rest quite comfortably at night knowing that should our food supply be totally cut off, I could nourish my children until they were through grade school and could forage for berries in the woods on their own.

So none of my clothes fit right. At the mall, I'd think about what I'd need to wear to an upcoming party and which stores I'd visit. Hours later I'd head home with a full trunk of—you guessed it: clothes for the baby. The thing about baby clothes is that they are all so adorable and would look especially adorable on my baby. I couldn't risk another baby wearing my baby's outfit, so I'd buy them all.

At the party I would make sure my conversation was especially scintillating, hoping no one would notice I was wearing my lime-green prom dress. Being 100 percent polyester, it was stretchy enough to fit over my hips, and this time the top fit without the benefit of a padded bra.

I've been a mom for ten years as of this month. I've recovered my old body. I don't have a baby to shop for anymore, but now I don't have time to shop. The good news is my lime-green prom dress is back in style. And I took the blue-and-white striped one and made a canopy for our beach trip this month.

Jan Butsch

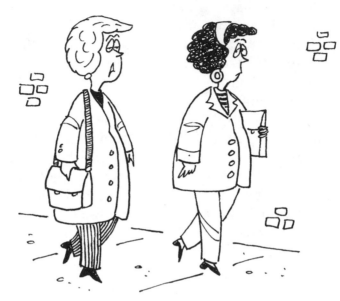

DAVE CARPENTER...

"Jennifer, the term 'blissfully pregnant'
is an oxymoron."

Hair Raising

As a young lieutenant's wife in the 1970s, I quickly learned that being "in the Army" was a whole-family experience. Many of the officers' wives served as volunteers on post, particularly the hospital.

During one checkup, when I was pregnant with my second child, the handsome doctor had difficulty pushing the sliding shelf at the end of the examining table back into the table. The two volunteers, both officers' wives, tried to help, but the doctor finally had to get down on his knees and keep the shelf level while pushing to remedy this problem. In the meantime, I suddenly felt something similar to a Brillo pad, brush my foot, which was on the stirrup. It became quickly apparent that this was no pot scrubber I felt on my foot, but the hairpiece, that moments before adorned the doctor's head! As he pulled away, his toupee was left hanging precisely from my little toe. He quickly snatched the hairpiece off my toe and placed it back on his head without a word.

Later that month, I was having coffee with other wives who volunteered at the hospital. Someone asked how I liked working at the Army hospital. I began laughing and shared my story about the toupee.

I admit I found it very embarrassing at the time, but hilarious later. As I finished my story, several of the women immediately grabbed their purses and began handing money to the others. It seems there was a long-standing bet among these women about whether this physician, indeed, wore a toupee. Several of them left that day with smiles on their faces and money in their pockets. The cat was out of the bag.

Susan Everett

Excerpted with permission from Belly Laughs and Babies, *compiled by Mary Sheridan* ©1997 *Laughing Stork Press.*

A Mother's Journey

My life forever changed on the day you were conceived,
Your heartbeat gave me the reality of what I had achieved.
The stages of your development, the picture of how you
grew,
Never completely knowing if I should buy in pink or blue.
Then came the day when I was able to hold you in my arms,
Hoping, as any mother would, to protect you against harm.
A precious little baby with ten tiny new toes,
An amazing set of lungs and a cute little button nose.
As you grow with lightning speed, I promise to treasure
every day,
And try my best to give you a rainbow when the sky is
dark and grey.

Elizabeth Butera

Expectant-ness

What I remember most about the months before my daughter's arrival was the "expectant-ness" with which I lived my life. There was the good expectant-ness, associated with the knowledge that we were about to adopt a beautiful baby girl who would forever alter the lives of my husband, my two sons and myself.

This was the one I cherished.

Then, there was the not-so-good expectant-ness, associated with the knowledge that my mother, diagnosed with terminal cancer and clinging to her final few months on this earth, would probably not live to meet her new granddaughter—a granddaughter for whom she had hoped and dreamed years before.

This was the one I dreaded.

Unbelievably, it was the mingling of these two kinds of expectant-ness which helped me understand the true meaning of "expecting."

I had received the call from my oldest sister, Linda, earlier that week, telling me that our mother was in the hospital again. It didn't look good, she whispered. Maybe I should come now, over the Thanksgiving holiday, to see her. I was torn. I had already flown home, to Indiana, from

Texas several times that year to see her, and my sons, ages five and seven, were looking forward to a chance to stay home this holiday. My husband, Brian, was also weary of traveling, but he understood the predicament in which I found myself.

"Go home," he said that night. "The boys and I will be just fine here. You need to be with your mom."

When I arrived at the hospital the next day, I could see that my sisters had not exaggerated. Mom smiled at me weakly from her bed.

"It must be bad if you returned from the sunny South," she murmured. I shrugged and joked about avoiding cooking a Thanksgiving turkey. We both settled into a comfortable silence, interrupted periodically by beeping and clicking of the I.V. machine in the corner. Finally, Mom spoke.

"Tell me all about the little girl." Her eyes, overcast and dull, brightened momentarily. So did mine, I know, as I filled her in on the four-month-old baby who, sight unseen, had seized our hearts. We talked for what seemed like hours, Mom sharing her memories of the four little girls she had brought into the world. She talked about how fun it was to dress all of us and brush our hair, to share feminine wisdom and secrets. And then we were quiet again, the room swollen with the expectant-ness of a new mother and an old one, about to retire her position forever.

The doctor released her to my sister's home the next day, knowing there was little more he could do for her there. She had been patched up with another blood transfusion, enough to get her through the turkey and cranberry sauce, and maybe a few days besides, before her blood would again begin to fail her. We all made it through the holiday with false cheeriness, and then returned to the business of sitting around and waiting—the business of expectant-ness.

A day or two later, my mother interrupted the terrible silences of the house.

"Have you bought much for the baby yet?"

I shook my head. I was an adoptive mother, having been through the state system with our sons. Our daughter would also be coming through the foster care system, and even though our experience before had been very positive, we knew better than to count on adoption paperwork always going according to plan. The less I purchased for the baby, the more secure I felt in her arrival. Call it one of those protective quirks that adoptive parents learn early on.

Mom smiled weakly, and Linda sat up straighter in her chair. "Hey! There's a baby-clothing outlet that just opened nearby! Let's go shopping!"

I hesitated. Should I explain my superstitions about shopping too early for the baby? Did I need to tell them how I was trying to protect myself, not wanting to have to bundle little pink dresses and blankets into boxes, bound for the attic, never to be used?

"That sounds like fun," Mom said quietly. I watched her eyes brighten. "Little pink dresses and booties and receiving blankets . . ."

It didn't take us long to load up her wheelchair and hit the road. We laughed and talked all the way there, remembering all the shopping trips we had taken before, the bargains we had found, the lunches over which we had lingered, the chocolate sodas with which we'd end our days. This was to be our final shopping trip, a mother and her daughters, filled with expectant-ness, for the day, and the promise of a new shopping companion, not yet arrived.

Mom swung into action immediately, her hands, bruised from the myriad of I.V. needles, reaching for pastel dresses with satin ribbons and flowers at the hem. She "oohed" and "aahed" over fluffy, pink blankets and hooded bath towels and caressed the brims of frilly hats, imagining, I suppose, the soft smell of the baby's head that would soon fill them. She directed my sister and me all over the store from her wheelchair perch, pointing to tiny washcloths and patterned sleepers. The life in her eyes buoyed me and carried me from my feeling of despair. I was an expectant mother, she bragged to every salesclerk in the store. We were going to have a baby girl in the family, and she would need to be dressed to the nines.

We went home that night and pulled our soft, pink treasures from a sea of bags that covered the living room floor. I watched my mother's watery eyes travel over each tiny outfit, and then light on me with a smile. The torch had been passed.

My daughter, Ellie, arrived two months later, three weeks after my mother finally lost her fight with cancer. I wrapped my baby lovingly in each of those beautiful dresses, and remembered that last shopping trip with my mother that showed me the real meaning of expectantness. On that day, I learned that expecting is more than waiting for something to happen. On that day, it was about living in the moments between.

Barbara Warner

3

FOR EXPECTANT FATHERS

Rose says that this is the day. I am dubious. After all, there have been no clarion cries from the heaven, no storks seen fleeting against the still wintery sky. It's much too ordinary a day for such a remarkable event as the birth of our baby.

Martin Paule

A Crash Course
in Epidurals and Diapers

Though actors are often wary during interviews, most turn instantly sincere on the subject of children, as Kevin Bacon did recently when he offered free advice to an expecting father.

"You know, there are hundreds of books for women about what to expect when you're expecting, or what to expect in the first year, but nothing for men. We are flying blind."

This is true. Jake Thompson arrived two weeks ago, and I can confirm that from Dad's point of view, the pregame literature is fairly incomplete, particularly on the crucial topic of delivery.

Since this is still fresh in my mind, allow me to fill in important gaps in the "What to Expect" canon.

You should know, for instance, that after such well-known unpleasantness as gigantic epidural needles and pushing and cursing and various other things that shall go politely unnamed, I saw an exasperated medical staff suddenly attack my wife with a giant vacuum cleaner.

At least it looked like a vacuum. I asked what it was. They said, "It's a vacuum." With a hose attachment that goes on the baby's head. I remember thinking that if the Three Stooges were doctors, this is what they'd try.

Later, I went back to the literature and checked, and could find no mention of this procedure. At no time during ten hours of childbirth classes did anyone mention that if pushing didn't work, the door would burst open and a team would rush in dragging a Hoover portable, which the doctor would use in an attempt to suck the baby out of Mommy.

Having seen the vacuum in action, several times, I understand why it's glossed over in the books and birthing classes—if people knew about it, they'd never go to the hospital.

For one thing, when you see the vacuum and the hose, and you weigh them against the three hours of strenuous pushing that has preceded their appearance, you'd guess there isn't a chance in hell it's going to work. And you'd be right.

Looking back, I'd say the real purpose of the vacuum is to make your child's head look like a Hershey's Kiss, which is what happened to Jake, who, at nearly nine pounds, wasn't going to come out at the urging of some glorified dust buster.

So it was on to surgery, where Jake got the luxury item accorded to all stubborn babies—a womb with a view. With a cesarean section, Dad, you have about ten minutes to confront the fact that all of your training now counts for nothing.

You are probably disoriented. The hospital uses this period of confusion to get you into a clown outfit—a great billowy shower cap, baggy shirt, puffy slippers and pants that barely cover your knees. Thus stripped of your dignity, you are herded into the operating room, where your wife is displayed on a table like some hapless volunteer in a magician's act, bisected by a curtain.

Watch us pull a baby out of your wife, even as she remains awake!

And sure enough, there's the physician, standing over her with cutting tools. My advice, fellas, is to concentrate on your spouse, who will be wide awake and looking to you for reassurance. Whatever you do, don't tell her what's going on behind the curtain and try not to look too closely when the nurse tells you the baby is being "extracted."

If you do sneak a peek, be advised that you will probably not want to eat a London broil for, oh, three to four years.

Also, forget those scenes from the movies, wherein the scruffy newborn is placed in the arms of his mother. Mom is still having her abdomen rearranged, so the nurse brings the baby straight to you.

And there your are, cradling an infant, doing something useful like singing "Row, Row, Row Your Boat," in the middle of an operating room where people are putting staples into your wife.

This is where you really have to remember your main job, which is holding it together. Because amid the chaos, the clatter of instruments, the casual medical babble ("Hey, look at this fibroid!"), your wife's wacky drug-induced monologue, the baby will suddenly stop crying and look right at you, and you realize, all of a sudden, that he knows your voice.

Watch out for that one.

From there, you get a well-deserved break. Your wife gets a bedroom, and if she's had a C-section, you get most of her food. This is Easy Street. Enjoy your last stroll.

When Baby is crying, you ship him across the hall to the nursery. When Baby needs changing, a helpful nurse is there to do it for you. At first. Gradually they invite you into the diaper-changing process, because they know what's coming, and you don't.

Meconium. Think of it as diaper shock therapy. God has decreed that one of baby's first bowel movements will be his most ungodly—an amount of roofing tar sufficient to re-shingle most five-bedroom homes.

This is nothing like the more innocuous movements to follow, though these make up in frequency what they lack in individual volume. Don't worry, they have stuff for this.

At our house, where we are creating a new pagan theology built around the twin deities of Grill Master and Thigh Master, we have gratefully added a new figure, Diaper Genie. He makes dirty diapers disappear.

Beneficent Diaper Genie is part of the essential modern baby-equipment package that also includes portable cradles, swivel seats, strollers that morph into other things, musical swinging chairs. They take only seven months to assemble, and cost no more than five million dollars.

But, as veteran fathers keep reminding me—it's all worth it.

Because when you come home at the end of the day, the little guy is waiting for you. He's resting in the crook of your arm, staring up with those big, luminous eyes and wearing a little grin that can only mean one thing.

He's just pooped in your hands.

Gary Thompson

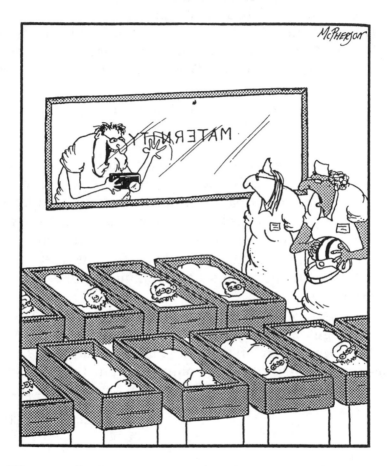

"That goofball over there offered me five bucks to put this helmet on his kid long enough to get a photo."

Father Hens

I could not point to any need in childhood as strong as that for a father's protection.

Sigmund Freud

The night after we brought our first child home from the hospital, I held him in the streetlight half-darkness of our living room. Joshua was crying, a little pink bird, his breath ragged, his arms and legs stretching aimlessly. I sang him an old Irish tune and found Mackey—from the Gaelic word for son.

In those first moments of fatherhood, I imagined all the daring acts I would perform in my boy's defense, all the intruders I would subdue. I laughed, noticing with a shiver the contrast between my dark fantasies and the perfect sweet-soft boy I cradled. As he fell asleep, a smudge of yawn and mew, I thought about my own father and a legacy that has made its way into my heart.

My father was a mother hen. Though it was my mother who raised the seven of us and did the thousand daily chores the brood demanded, it was my father's job to worry about us. For him, it was an article of faith that life was out to get us kids, that no creatures as fine as his children could be safe in this brutal world.

He came by his concern honestly. He was a doctor, a general practitioner with a thriving practice. He saw the dreadful things that couldn't possibly happen to children, except that they did. He warned us about lawn mowers, diving boards, lighter fluid, fish hooks, hunks of steak, "projectiles" of all sorts. He warned us about traffic, doors, windows and ice. He told us cautionary tales about broken bones, sledding accidents, a boy killed on a horse. A garrulous, cheerful man, he was also a connoisseur of chaos.

When our son was born, my wife and I began baby-proofing our apartment. We bought caps for outlets, cushions for sharp corners. We locked closets, installed gates, stashed matches, checked the floor for splinters. We even checked the ceiling for splinters.

And then we waited as Josh blossomed into danger, lifting his head, rolling over, crawling. Finally he stood up and walked, a staggering little drunk with a rabbit on his shirt. Suddenly he was tall enough to bang his head on the dining-room table, then nimble enough to scramble over a chair. Each accomplishment brought new peril. I thought we would never be able to protect him. Once when he was six months old I had a dream about him. We were caught in a lightning storm, and I saw myself crouching over Josh, pleading with the sky.

About lightning, my father was a poet of doom. We were not only to come inside at the first drop of rain, but we were also to stay away from windows. According to Dad, no prudent person even took a shower when it was raining. When my brother Kevin and I were teenagers, Dad once drove his car across a golf course to scoop us up from the fourteenth green. We thought Mom had died. Not so. Dad had heard a weather report that rain was on the way.

Dad was a genius in his caution. Yes, we had to agree, it was not impossible to choke on a croquet mallet, and yes, though we'd never heard of anybody suffocating in a baseball mitt, we supposed that, too, could happen.

About driving, he was a master. Statistics had proved that there were more drunk drivers on the road on Sunday afternoon than at any other time of the week. Or perhaps it was during Lent, or when it was hot—he would customize his warnings to fit each situation. As for sleeping over at friends' houses, he was a stickler. He wanted his kids home.

He did, however, make one exception. When Kevin and I were Boy Scouts, we asked, with little hope, if we could go on a canoe trip. My father replied with all sorts of questions: What adults were going? How long would it last? We answered in reassuring tones, awaiting his inevitable response: more Irish-Catholic boys died on canoe trips than in World War II.

Suddenly he got up and called the Scoutmaster, asking questions, greeting each response with a skeptical grunt. Hanging up, he rubbed his hands in excitement. "Good news, boys," he chirped. "I'm going with you. The O'Neils hit the Great White North."

We couldn't believe it. We wondered if Dad knew that camping meant sleeping outside, the place where it rained. Where bears lived. We arrived at the lake, convinced the sight of water would remind Dad that most people died of drowning. But no. We set out into the setting orange sun, a string of canoes, each loaded with two boys and a man. That night we pitched tents, cooked burgers, put on sweaters against the October chill and fell asleep, canvas-covered and little-boy-bone-tired in the grip of an adventure.

Morning came cold and wet. Bundled in sweaters and rain gear, we set off across the lake. We were the last

canoe in the chain, and the wind made the lake tough
going. Before long, as the fog grew thick and the wind
beat the water into a gray-white chop, we lost sight of the
rest of the boats. From the stern came, "Let's catch up,
boys," and I laid my eighty-two pounds heartily into the
paddle. Suddenly a wave hit the canoe broadside, over-
turning it, and dropping us into the frigid lake. We were
a few hundred yards from a small island. As I came bob-
bing up, I thought this was going to be a great adventure.
But when I saw my father, his hair soaked crazily to his
head, his face a white mask, I knew this was no adventure. That remains the only time I have ever seen him
scared. He glanced at me and looked quickly around.
"Kev-in!" he barked.

"I'm over here, Dad," Kevin said from the far side of the
overturned canoe. "I'm all right."

"Hang on to the boat, boys," Dad said calmly. "I'm
going to push it to the island."

"Why don't we just swim, Dad?" I asked.

"Hang on to the boat, Hugh!" he shouted like a stranger.

Dad struggled with the clumsy canoe, and it began to
move toward the island, saddled with two shivering
forms, a submarine now, headed for landfall. Suddenly,
my father let out a giant roar. "Help! Help!" It scared me.
"Help," he shouted again.

"They didn't hear . . ." Kevin began.

"Quiet!" Dad yelled, and as his voice caromed off the
wind, an engine snarled to life, yapping across the water
toward us. Finally the shape emerged from the fog, one
man standing up in the bow, a second one crouched over
an outboard motor—a gray presence coming out of a
muted white morning sun. They fished us out of the
water.

"Don't worry now, boys. You're okay."

When we got to the island, the men started a bonfire.

Dad took off all his clothes, told us to do the same, and we stood next to the blaze, three naked heathens. I remember its heat coming at me in great thumping waves. I remember my father wrapping his arms around us—rubbing our hands, our arms, our feet, our hearts. "Thank you, fellas," he said to the men across the flames. "You saved my boys."

When I was sixteen my father's caution began to drive me crazy. Here I was taxiing for takeoff and he had his arms around my ankles. I used to imagine the romantic lives my friends led—letting the wind whip through their windows, staying out till all hours, taking showers in all kinds of weather.

Now, from my new-parent perspective, Dad's caution makes sense. In fact, I occasionally wonder whether my father wasn't a bit cavalier. After all, he let me play Little League baseball, a game in which an oversized twelve-year-old throws a rock-hard sphere with as much velocity as possible toward your child.

As parents, we want it both ways. We want our kids to know all the world's exhilarating stuff. But we want them to learn about it in a padded room down the hall. And this feeling never ends. Not long ago we shared a rented beach house with my brother and his family, and our parents came to visit us. As Kevin and I bounded around the surf, riding the waves on our bellies, I looked up and saw my mother and father walking along the water's edge, trying to look casual, but gesturing for us to come in, and finally shouting across the wind to their grown sons, "Boys, don't go out too far!"

Though I talk to my father rarely these days, he is never far away. Recently, my wife and I were planning to escape on our first childless vacation, and I heard myself suggesting that we take separate planes. If we did, although the chance of Josh's losing one parent was doubled, the chance of his losing both virtually disappeared. After thanking me for a cheerful start to our vacation, Jody recognized my father's style.

"Did your parents fly separately?" she asked.

"No," I answered. "They stayed home."

Hugh O'Neil

Deep in Dadland

Greetings to all my friends . . .

I am sending this e-mail to you to let you know that I am okay. Don't give away my spot on the end of the bar at Charlie's or get anyone else to play third base on the team just yet. I'll be back. I just don't know when.

The reason you haven't heard from me lately is that I've been hiding out in a plastic fort behind my garage. There's a small but spirited band of three- to six-year-olds that are looking for me at the moment. A couple of them even belong to me. I tried to interest them in hide-and-seek, but they wanted to play "Vaporize the Alien" instead. Guess who was voted in as the Alien.

That was weeks ago. I had no idea how obsessive kids are today. I'm kind of lucky they've been mostly playing spaceship with the cardboard box this fort came in. They're not that much smarter than we were at their age. But they definitely have better cash flow.

I'm a full-time dad now. If one more person calls me Mr. Mom, or tells me "I look like I have my hands full," I'm going to spit up on them. This isn't temporary. Believe me, I don't miss work. I can't. I work harder now than I ever did at my job. No sick days. No Monday-morning water-cooler sessions. No casual trips to the office coffee pot. As most of you probably know, I spent the last few years at my old job toiling away at basically meaningless work in an inhospitable environment, drowning my creative self in mind-numbing routine. Most jobs I've had were like that. Except this one.

I was trying to hollow out a small cave of competency in a sand dune of stupidity, armed with only a plastic spoon and a Barney Rubble sip cup filled with gin. The sand dune won. Here I am today. My left leg is fast asleep. It's been in a full upright and locked position since last Thursday.

The first kid is easy. You start researching fine cigars. You practice your juggling. You have nine months to paint a room (whoa!), learn how to coach your wife to breathe (duh), and read a couple of articles about diapering techniques and time-outs in magazines with cute bald babies on the cover. How hard is that? Everyone treats you like you won the lottery. Congratulations! You've just been upgraded to Dad status! You're in the Dad Club! You get to shop in a whole new aisle at the grocery store, one you've never even *seen* before.

When the second child comes along (and the third— after that, who's counting?) is when you really find out what you're in for. That's where I'm at now. To be fair, I wasn't drafted for this duty. I enlisted on my own free will. I just didn't realize how long boot camp was going to last.

On the positive side, I think our baby, Bartholomew, is a genius. He has a vocabulary that is expanding at a remarkable rate. Today, at the age of only three months, we're pretty sure he can speak about four languages and six dialects. We've contacted an early language and linguistics expert to identify which ones they are exactly, since to our untrained ears he sounds like either an extremely intoxicated bull elephant seal or a screech owl giving birth to a basketball.

Our other boys are doing well too. Kevin is busy renaming the Seven Dwarfs for a kindergarten thesis project and drawing their pictures: Sticky, Icky, Greasy, Motley, Chewy, Hairball and Spud. He's going to present the drawings to us at his graduation ceremony that's coming up. Give me a break. Graduation from kindergarten? With caps and gowns and everything? Frankly, I think this self-esteem thing is out of hand.

Joey, our younger boy, is delving into a craft project his mother found in one of those magazines I mentioned earlier. He's packing leftover baby rice cereal mash into old ice cube trays and baking them into bricks in the hot sun. He wants to build an outdoor adobe play hut for himself and his action figures to live in full time. The doctors say he's making progress. We have our fingers crossed.

But hey. Fatherhood is rewarding. Really. It's truly a beautiful experience when you kneel on a tiny plastic block while playing "horsey" for two. (Maybe that's where the baby's learning all of those new vocabulary words.) Or the wonders of storytime . . . spending an hour putting the kids to sleep with about a billion stories about lost bunnies and lonely balloons, only to wake them up by stepping on a talking Pooh book in the dark and having to start over. Or finding a banana that died of exposure behind the living-room sofa. Or the cordless telephone in the dog's water bowl. I could go on. They're right when they say it's getting to be a small world after all.

As you can probably tell, I'm spending a lot of time with the kids. I'm learning new stuff every day, even about my house itself. The only part I was familiar with before was the backyard and maybe the garage. Now I'm on a first-name basis with every room, mostly because I have to clean them three to four times an hour. My kitchen appliances are not just machines to me anymore. They have personalities, quirks, tendencies, even habits.

I think I've passed over some kind of threshold. I went to an open house at the preschool with a Batman sticker on my shoulder. A strange woman with a bemused smile gently plucked it off me, with the same gesture she probably uses to brush dandruff off her husband's cardigan or wipe peanut butter from her toddler's cheek. We all laughed politely and that was that. I didn't really mind. She had cracker crumbs in her hair.

Oops . . . gotta go. I think I hear the pitter-patter of little feet. E-mail me back with word from the outside if you get a chance. I'm not going anywhere. I've got eighteen years or so to wait. So far, so good.

T. Brian Kelly

THE FAMILY CIRCUS　　　**By Bil Keane**

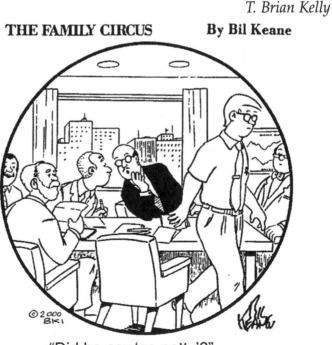

"Did he say 'go potty'?"

Reprinted by permission of Bil Keane.

Love Letters

Steve had been a dedicated labor coach. In Lamaze class, he held my head gently and panted along with me. He learned the names of all the different types of breathing and memorized the order in which I was to do them. I didn't have to think; my job, he said, was just to lay back and deliver the baby. He was cool, he was in control; two qualities I found comforting since I wasn't sure what to expect with our first child.

A couple of weeks before I was due, I had two T-shirts made; one for Steve that said, "Coach," and another for our soon-to-be-born infant that said "Assistant Coach." The baby's shirt was so tiny that the letters covered all but the neck and sleeves. Steve didn't hesitate to try his on. "Now you're official," I said with a grin.

All through my pregnancy, I had heard stories of men who empathized with their wives' conditions so strongly that they would put on an additional thirty pounds or feel phantom heart flutters. Steve never showed that kind of emotional tie to my experience. He was happy and proud but wanted to stay calm so he could help me. That's why I never expected what happened the night I delivered.

I had been timing my contractions since midday, and in

my mind, there was no doubt what was happening. So when Steve came home from work about 9 P.M., I simply said, "We have to go to the hospital. Now."

"Now?" he said with his head in the refrigerator, searching for the makings of a sandwich.

"Now!" I said, holding my belly as another pressure wave rolled through.

"Has your water broken yet?" he asked matter-of-factly as he smeared mustard on his bread.

"No, but the contractions are already starting. Let's go."

"Hand me a pen," he said, cool as the cucumbers he was now eating. He took a notepad out of his pocket. "Tell me when you get the next one."

I wrote two columns on the paper; one that said "Time" and the other that said "Length." I made the first notation, because he was still eating. I saw him jot down three more before he said, "Okay. Maybe you've got something here. I'll drive you over to the hospital and we'll see."

The rest of the night was something of a blur for me. I labored, I pushed, and by dawn, we had a beautiful new daughter in our arms. What I didn't know is that I wasn't the only one giving birth. Mr. "cool, calm and collected" had lived every moment with me, keeping extensive notes of everything that happened.

When I awakened the next morning, Steve handed me six sheets of paper and our new daughter's journal. On the papers was my one notation of my contractions, followed by the recording of more than fifty others. Steve's neat, precise handwriting became looser and obviously more fatigued as the night wore on. Although I slept between contractions, he had not, keeping a silent, steady vigil so as not to miss anything. He chronicled every word he or anyone else said during my admittance. Although he obviously tried to create an objective record of the experience, his own emotions came shining through every line. I could see that he was laboring right along with me as he struggled to keep his surgical mask on his face while trying to keep up with my every breath. Every other sentence ended with an exclamation point as his wonder and excitement built. In almost every way, he was much more aware of the event than I was, and much more awed by the result. "I was the first to shout, 'It's a girl!'" he wrote. All I could remember thinking was, *What a relief to be able to stop pushing!*

I looked over at him. Sometime during the night, he had changed into his "Coach" T-shirt. Together, we put the "Assistant Coach" T-shirt on our new daughter, which hung down to her pretty little pink toes. The real love letters, however, were not the ones emblazoned across his chest or hers but the ones he handed to me, which will have a treasured place in my heart forever.

Robin Silverman

The Mercedes

There's nothing like a new car in the neighborhood to bring the guys together.

"Nice car, Wayne," I said.

Mike crossed over from his house: "Hey Wayne, new or used?"

"Used."

John was two steps behind Mike. "Six or eight cylinders?"

"Four."

Jim peeked over the fence: "CD or cassette?"

"Neither."

We were all impressed. Then, the new neighbor appeared out of nowhere and stole Wayne's moment.

"Wow, look at that!"

We stared, our mouths dropped open, as Bob Henderson parked his new Mercedes in his driveway. We watched him walk inside.

"No kids, you know," Mike said breaking the silence.

"Probably waiting until they've gone through their selfish stage."

"Yeah," we chimed. We had enough kids amongst us to field our own Little League team—bat boy included.

Jim pointed to the Mercedes. "Imagine owning a

beautiful car like that with no one kicking the back of your seat."

"Ever notice how baby formula cuts through new car smell faster than a toddler passes salsa?"

"Yeah," we said.

"I saw his wife and him going out again last night. All dressed up."

"Must be nice not paying for a baby-sitter."

"We received a lovely card the other day from our sitter thanking us for the 401K and profit-sharing plan."

"He leaves early and comes home late from work any time he wants."

"Wives only want us around for crowd control."

"Yeah," we chanted.

"I bet his watch doesn't get buried in the backyard like treasure."

"I doubt he's ever worked all day oblivious to a Barbie sticker on his butt."

"He can eat his dinner while it's hot."

"And not standing up."

"Yeah," we said, standing there shaking our heads.

Wayne's wife brought out a tray of lemonade. "What are you guys staring at?"

Wayne gestured across the street: "The neighbors' new car, we were just saying if they had kids it . . ."

"They can't have children, you know," she announced.

The five of us looked at each other.

"They're infertile." She passed out the lemonade and returned to the house. Except for the tinkling of ice against the glasses, it was quiet for a long time.

"It's a nice car, Wayne."

"I think I'll go see what my kids are doing."

"Yeah."

Ken Swarner

Daddy's Girl

As I button the last button on her frilly new dress, she reminds me, "Don't forget to poof up the sleeves, Mom." Finally with sleeves perfectly inflated, and slip, tights and patent-leather shoes all in their proper places, she dashes off to the full-length mirror to admire herself. "It's the prettiest dress in the whole world, isn't it, Mom."

"You bet," I respond. This is the night of the Father/Daughter Dance, and we've been looking forward to it for weeks.

"This is gonna be better than Christmas, almost!" She giggles as I ready her hair for the fancy ribbon.

I imagine her dancing the night away with her Prince Charming—Dad. My mind drifts back to the image of this child who didn't have a Daddy until after she could say the word. My husband Ron, handsome, middle-aged, told the caseworker, "It doesn't matter to me if it's a boy or a girl."

Months later, on short notice, we flew from Ohio to Seattle with our two other children in tow. That night we hardly slept a wink in our hotel room.

The next morning, eager to meet the new addition to our family, we arrived at the adoption agency offices before they opened for the day. It seemed like hours until

finally, Susie, our daughter's birth mother, walked in holding each of Elaina's hands to guide her. Elaina took one
look at Ron and shouted, "Da-Da."

That was it. Hearts melted as he scooped her up in his
big arms to say hello. I didn't know who I wanted to hug
first, Elaina or her birth mother.

Susie was so brave to make this decision. She'd had an
adoption plan in place when she was pregnant with
Elaina. But when the birth father came to the hospital saying they should get back together to raise their child, she
hoped it would work. It didn't. A few months later Susie
was alone again, going to school, working and trying to
raise Elaina. She did the best she could, but after nearly a
year, she realized that she wanted more for her daughter.
She wanted Elaina to be raised with a mommy, daddy and
siblings. She happened upon the agency we were working with and chose us from a family picture book we had
submitted.

As soon as we met her, I felt an immediate bond to
Susie. It's that everlasting bond of motherhood we share
because of our love for Elaina.

Susie has gone on to school and kept in touch with us
for a while. I know that even if we never hear from her
again she'll always be a part of our lives.

As I dab a bit of lipstick on our little girl's lips, Dad
emerges from the bedroom. He's dressed in his navy pin-
striped suit and brightly colored animal tie that Elaina
gave him for his last birthday. He takes one look at Elaina
and exclaims "Wowee, you look beautiful, Princess!"

I know he's nearly as excited as she is. Tonight there's
magic in the air. Tonight Elaina's Daddy will experience
the thrill of his daughter riding on his feet as they swirl
across the dance floor. They'll share such delicacies as
macaroni and cheese, pizza and hot dogs, while joining in
the Limbo and Hokey Pokey.

As they head out the door, she stops one more time for a quick glance in the mirror. "I really do look like a princess, don't I, Dad?"

As his eyes meet mine, they tell me we're both thinking what we've talked about before. Nothing compares to the love between a little girl and her daddy.

Nancy M. Surella

This Is My Son

To understand your parents' love, you must raise children of your own.

Chinese Proverb

This is 1963.

From deep in the canyoned aisles of a supermarket comes what sounds like a small-scale bus wreck followed by an air raid. If you followed the running box-boy armed with mop and broom, you would come upon a young father, his three-year-old son, an upturned shopping cart and a good part of the pickles shelf—all in a heap on the floor.

The child, who sits on a plastic bag of ripe tomatoes, is experiencing what might nicely be described as "significant fluid loss." Tears, mixed with mucus from a runny nose, mixed with blood from a small forehead abrasion, mixed with saliva drooling from a mouth that is wide open, and making a noise that would drive a dog under a bed. The kid has also wet his pants and will likely throw up before this little tragedy reaches bottom. He has that "stand back, here it comes" look of a child in a pre-urp condition. The small lake of pickle juice surrounding the child doesn't make rescue any easier for the supermarket 911 squad arriving on the scene.

The child is not hurt. And the father has had some experience with the uselessness of the stop-crying-or-I'll-smack-you syndrome and has remained amazingly quiet and still in the face of the catastrophe.

The father is calm because he is thinking about running away from home. Now. Just walking away, getting into the car, driving away somewhere down South, changing his name, getting a job as a paperboy or a cook in an all-night diner. Something—anything—that doesn't involve contact with three-year-olds.

Oh sure, someday he may find all this amusing, but in the most private part of his heart he is sorry he has children, sorry he married, sorry he grew up, and, above all, sorry that this particular son cannot be traded in for a model that works. He will not and cannot say these things to anybody, ever, but they are there and they are not funny.

The box-boy and the manager and the accumulated spectators are terribly sympathetic and consoling. Later, the father sits in his car in the parking lot holding the sobbing child in his arms until the child sleeps. He drives home and carries the child up to his crib and tucks him in. The father looks at the sleeping child for a long time. The father does not run away from home.

This is 1976.

Same man paces my living room, carelessly cursing and weeping by turns. In his hand is what's left of a letter that has been crumpled into a ball and then uncrumpled again several times. The letter is from his sixteen-year-old son (same son). The pride of his father's eye—or was until today's mail.

The son says he hates him and never wants to see him again. The son is going to run away from home. Because of his terrible father. The son thinks the father is a failure as a parent. The son thinks the father is a jerk.

What the father thinks of the son right now is somewhat incoherent, but it isn't nice.

Outside the house it is a lovely day, the first day of spring. But inside the house it is more like *Apocalypse Now*, the first day of one man's next stage of fathering. The old gray ghost of Oedipus has just stomped through his life. Someday—some long day from now—he may laugh about even this. For the moment there is only anguish.

He really is a good man and a fine father. The evidence of that is overwhelming. And the son is quality goods as well. Just like his father, they say. "Why did this happen to me?" the father shouts at the ceiling.

Well, he had a son. That's all it takes. And it doesn't do any good to explain about that right now. First you have to live through it. Wisdom comes later. Just have to stand there like a jackass in a hailstorm and take it.

This is 1988.

Same man and same son. The son is twenty-eight now, married, with his own three-year-old son, home, career and all the rest. The father is fifty.

Three mornings a week I see them out jogging together around 6:00 A.M. As they cross a busy street, I see the son look both ways, with a hand on his father's elbow to hold him back from the danger of oncoming cars, protecting him from harm. I hear them laughing as they run on up the hill into the morning. And when they sprint toward home, the son doesn't run ahead but runs alongside his father at his pace.

They love each other a lot. You can see it.

The are very careful of each other—they have been through a lot together, but it's all right now.

One of their favorite stories is about once upon a time in a supermarket.

This is Now.

And this story is always. It's been lived thousands of times, over thousands of years, and literature is full of examples of tragic endings, including that of Oedipus. The sons leave, kick away and burn all bridges, never to be seen again. But sometimes (more often than not, I suspect) they come back in their own way and in their own time and take their own fathers in their arms. That ending is an old one, too. The father of the Prodigal Son could tell you.

Robert Fulghum

I've Never Been So Scared

Love is the true means by which the world is enjoyed: our love to others, and others' love to us.

Thomas Traherne

Dear Blair,

Happy birthday! It's hard to believe that my daughter is three years old today. "My daughter" . . . those words mean so much to me.

I wanted to give you a special present today. So I'm sharing with you some thoughts I jotted down three years ago while I was on a plane, flying to California to pick you and Mom up, eternally grateful to your birth mother for letting us adopt you into our family. Your brother Max and I were thirty thousand feet above Nevada heading to Los Angeles. We were four hours into the flight from New York. Max, who was three and a half years old at the time, had finally fallen asleep. I looked at his face and felt the love that fathers have felt for their children since the beginning of time.

I was on my way to meet you, my new daughter, and your mother at a gate in Los Angeles International Airport.

I was so happy and so scared. You were two days old, and from what everyone had told me over the phone, you were quite beautiful. Without even meeting you I knew you were my daughter, and we would share a life together because of circumstances beyond our control.

I also knew you would have to deal with the fact that you are adopted, given to us by a birth mother and birth father, able to conceive children but unable to provide for them. I made a commitment to do everything in my power to explain the process of adoption to you in a way that would foster your growth as a woman and a person, and not as a victim.

Both your mother and I believe that God picked you for us because we have lessons to teach each other. Max, at three and a half, had already taught me valuable lessons about my ability to love, nurture—and what a gift it is to be called "Dad."

I'm not sure either of you children will ever realize just how wanted you really were. I am sure you will know how loved you are. I suppose some parents who adopt spoil their kids by smothering them with love. Knowing myself and your mom, that's a real possibility. Will you ever fully appreciate how many visits to infertility clinics, special examinations and miscarriages it took for us to realize that having a family—not a pregnancy—was what we wanted? Or about the morning when we understood beyond a shadow of a doubt that there were many ways to build a family, and all of them open doors into the parenthood club; the biological port is not the only entrance.

I doubt you and Max will realize how diligently your mother placed ads in small-town newspapers around the country, hoping to find a birth mother who would give a child a gift of life and us the ultimate gift of love. Will you ever completely know how each time our telephone rang, our hearts were in our throats because this could have been the call we had been waiting for? There was so much pressure just to say the right things to the birth mothers, not to sound too old, or too anxious or even too educated to the seventeen-year-old girl on the other end of the line. I'm not sure you will care about those days; I wonder if knowing about those days will ever be important to you and your brother.

Adoption has taught me much that I could never have learned without going through it: how there is only one definition of the words "father," "mother," "son," "daughter": someone who has the capacity to love any human being as their own.

That's why I was so scared. Back when you were born, two child custody cases had been in the news. One, Baby Jessica, involved a birth mother who changed her mind before the adoption was finalized. The courts took the child away from her adoptive parents and returned to her birth parents—people she did not know.

Another case returned a teenaged girl to her birth parents after the hospital discovered that, years earlier, two infants had been switched at birth. No one would have known except that one of the children became very sick and died; during her sickness, blood tests revealed that she could not be the biological child of the people raising her. The surviving teen was torn, against her will, from the only family she had ever known. Both cases gave parents (biological and adoptive) nightmares. And both cases reminded me that in some states the law does not look at the bonds between children and their parents as we think and feel they should.

Even as I watched these two cases unfold, I never doubted our decision to adopt. I admit, I wanted to ask the judges if either could give up a child he and his wife had loved as their own, a child they'd raised for thirteen years, two years, one year or even one month, just because she really was not their biological daughter? Could anyone? I doubt it.

That's the scary part of adoption in this great country of ours. There really is no way around the fact that until the adoption is finalized, the adoptive parents walk around waiting for someone to throw a wrench into the works. Fortunately, adoptions are reversed in only a very few cases. But those rare cases break real hearts, and strike terror in the souls of all who choose to adopt. Because once you hold a baby in your arms, the only thing you want to do is love and protect that child forever. You block out the fact that during the period it takes to finalize the adoption, one phone call can shatter your world.

As I was mulling these thoughts over in my mind, the steward announced that we were ten minutes from landing. I was minutes away from stepping off the airplane and meeting my new daughter, Max's new sister. I knew how I'd hug and kiss your mom, the mother of our two children. I'd brought a camera so we could take pictures, and was sure that we'd both start to cry. Slowly, I knew, my fears would subside. Over time, love conquers all, but right at that moment I was so scared. All I could hope was that no one had experienced a change of heart, or mind.

For now, Blair, I'm just thankful that the wait is over, and all went well. And while these words mean little to you today, I hope someday you'll be able to share them with children of your own. I want you to be able to say, with pride, that your family was built the way all families should be: from love. I want you to tell your children how much love their grandparents put into creating a family.

Happy birthday, daughter.

Love,

Dad

David E. Mittman

$\overline{4}$

CHALLENGES ALONG THE WAY

Before you were conceived I wanted you.
Before you were born I loved you.
Before you were here an hour I would die
* for you.*
This is the miracle of love.

Maureen Hawkins

The Baby's Stash

"How are we going to pay for the baby, Jim?" my wife Lois asked with concern in her voice. We had just received the news from the doctor about the upcoming birth of our first child. The news was met with joyful innocence, now reality was sinking in. I'm sure questions about birth expenses and how they will be paid are universal. They were in our case at least.

I had just started a new job and had only minimal medical insurance, Lois was only working part time and had no insurance whatsoever. "Don't worry Hon," I said with confidence, "I'll find a way." And indeed I did.

I paid for our first child with $2.00 bills. I was paid on a weekly basis and my employer paid in cash when you presented your timeslip. The even dollar amount from the last $10.00 or close to it was always paid in $2.00 bills. They did this so they could determine if you were spending anything in their establishment. Even then (late '50s) $2.00 bills were scarce, with few in normal circulation.

We had been told the doctor bill would be $150.00 and the hospital bill would be $175.00. This figure seemed like a lot to a guy making $58.50 a week, clear. What a difference forty-five years makes. The medical procedures have changed little but the monetary aspect of medical bills has become almost frightening. As the weeks progressed I would dutifully arrive home after each payday and hand Lois all my $2.00 bills.

She had created a secret hiding place in the cupboard where she kept our "Baby Stash" as she laughingly called it. I never knew where it was so I had no idea how much we were accumulating. Whenever I would ask she would only smile, point to her now protruding stomach and say, "You will have to ask the baby." I would just smile, pick up the evening paper and say, "He doesn't feel like talking tonight." You see I had already decided on the baby's gender. It's sort of a macho thing with males. Fortunately wives seem to understand.

As the weeks turned into months I knew our Baby Stash was growing almost as fast as the baby was. The funny thing is—I never missed the money because I knew the $2.00 bills were not mine to keep. Like all pregnancies the delivery day finally arrived.

Awakening in the middle of the night, I reached over for Lois and she was gone, leaving a warm spot where she should have been. Then I heard her in the front room. *What's that noise?* I thought to myself. *Sounds like she is ironing.* I raised up in bed and hollered to her, "What are you doing?" "Ironing," she said matter-of-factly. "What for?" I asked. "It's time to go to the hospital and I want my new dress smock to look freshly pressed. Get up. Grab the suitcase and go out and start the car." By the time our fourth child was born I knew this routine by heart. For you see it never changed. The only thing that changed was the manner we paid for our other children. Plus our cars were newer and easier to start.

Throughout the years I have progressed in my career and the other children were fully covered by medical insurance. I was glad for this fact and so was Lois but it was sad in a way. For you see medical insurance can't cover the surprised smile on a doctor's face when you hand him a fistful of $2.00 bills and say, "Here's your fee, Doctor." Nor can a check from the insurance company ever take the place of Lois's Baby Stash and the warm feeling we both shared when I handed her my weekly $2.00 bills.

I had forgotten about the forty-two-year-old episode in my life until recently. I was at the supermarket when a dirty, worn $2.00 bill was placed in my hand along with my change. A lump arose in my throat and tears came to my eyes as I gazed at its tattered corners. Our Baby's Stash and all it represented had arisen from my memory in a blinding flash.

Struggling with my groceries, along with my memories, I walked toward my car and headed home to an empty apartment. Turning into my driveway I reflected how much fun it would be to start a Baby Stash once again. Then reality set in. There isn't enough time left in my life or enough $2.00 bills in circulation any more. Then I grinned as I thought—maybe, just maybe I could start another Baby Stash using our new gold dollars—dreamer.

James A. Nelson

A Precious Gift

"Are you going to find out what it is?"

"Well, we're really hoping it's a baby, but I did see a lady on the front of the *Enquirer* who had kittens . . ." Okay, okay, so I never actually answered anyone like that, but I was tempted many times. By the time I entered my seventh month, I had already gotten used to ridiculous questions (e.g., "Haven't you had that baby yet?" or "Well, are you ready?" and the ever-popular, "Won't you be glad to have it?"). And since my husband and I had chosen not to learn the sex of our first child, we decided we would ask the sex of our second child at the seven-month ultrasound. We already had a happy, healthy four-year-old son, so our decision to find out invited many comments like a) "Maybe this one will be a girl," b) "Well, when you get that daughter you'll have the perfect family," or c) "Now Matt needs a sister." Although I secretly longed for a daughter I kept telling myself that it didn't really matter.

The morning of my ultrasound I was a nervous wreck. The doctor had told me to drink the requisite fourteen gallons of water and, the fool that I am, I followed her instructions. By the time we drove the thirty minutes to the office I was about to die, and after I waited in the reception area for another thirty minutes I was standing on the edge of hysterical. After all, hell hath no fury like a pregnant woman denied her right to potty. I begged them to let me go to the bathroom, but they gave me a tiny cup and said, "Just a little," with an unsympathetic smirk. I made a Herculean effort to stop my flow and went back to the waiting room. Finally, it was time for the test. After smearing incredibly cold gel on my swelling tummy, I was parked unceremoniously on my back on a cot. The tech strapped every possible monitor firmly (read: tightly!) around me and I began to wonder if I could ever feel any less attractive. Surely this is what a beached whale feels like. I fully expected a group of Greenpeace activists to break in, shouting, "Don't worry! We'll get you back in! You're gonna be fine, Shamu." She began to describe the flickering image on the screen. "I see the heart, and all ventricles appear perfectly formed. The brain also appears normal. Measuring the legs, we can determine the approximate weight to see if we're on track with your due date." Dramatic pause, and then the announcement. "And if you want to know the sex, I can definitely tell . . . it's a boy!"

Her lips kept moving after that, but I didn't catch too much of it. All I do remember is trying to maintain my composure while my husband held my four-year-old (who was squealing with delight). I am human enough to admit that I was disappointed at first. The drive home was the longest thirty minutes of my life. And after I closed the bedroom door, the tears finally came, bringing with them the acknowledgement that I didn't want a daughter so I could have "a boy and a girl, the perfect family," and I didn't want a daughter so my son could protect her at school. I wanted a daughter for me. I wanted a little girl to wear mother/daughter dresses with, to go to the hair salon with, to go shopping with (for prom dresses, wedding gowns) and to sniffle through *It's a Wonderful Life* with. And as I kept on thinking about it, I realized that my deeper desire was not for a daughter but to go back and do my adolescence again.

Then something happened that really changed my perspective for the good—the phone rang. Our dearest friends were calling to tell us she had gotten some bad news from her ob-gyn that same afternoon—she was in the same stage of pregnancy as I was—and she was experiencing some complications. We cried and prayed with them and for them, and as I hung up the phone I began to realize what an amazing gift of life was moving inside me.

As I drove to work the next morning I braced myself for the impending question, "Did you find out what it is?" And immediately I knew the answer: Yes, I do know what it is. It is a gift. It is life. It is a priceless treasure. It is healthy; it is whole. It is another chance. It is laughter; it is joy. It is part of me. It is my son.

Kelli S. Jones

My Unborn Baby Saved My Life

My husband and I were thrilled when I finally got pregnant after a year of trying. The winter's first snow covered our rhododendron bushes like a pure, downy baby's blanket. As I gazed out my bedroom window, I wondered if the baby growing inside me would love to make snow angels and watch crystallized flakes melt on his or her little mittens.

I was thirty-one, in the fifth month of my first pregnancy, feeling energetic and alive. Steve and I couldn't wait to be parents. The fertility drug I took had worked. We believed things were finally going our way.

I didn't, however, have time to daydream about the baby and go for a leisurely walk in the snow. As a television reporter for the CBS affiliate in Portland, Oregon, snow meant one thing to me: standing knee-deep in a drift with wet flakes blowing in my face as I warned viewers not to drive.

It happened as I dressed for work. Without warning, a sharp pain shot through my abdomen. I doubled over, then curled into a ball on the bed.

I managed to call Steve, who was already at work. "You've got to come home now," I gasped. "Something's really wrong with me." He immediately headed out into the gridlock rush hour traffic to get home.

As the pain continued to come in waves, I called my ob-gyn's office. "I'm in a lot of pain," I told the nurse, crying so hard by now that it was difficult to speak. "I'm afraid I'm going to lose the baby!"

"Take deep breaths and try to relax," the nurse said. "You need to come in so we can examine you. How soon can you be here?"

An hour later my husband and I were in the examining room with an ob-gyn, a radiologist and an ultrasound technician. The doctor and the radiologist watched intently, their faces revealing nothing as the ultrasound technician helped us make sense of the hazy black-and-white images. There were plenty of things to see: heart valves pumping away and a beautiful facial profile right down to the little button nose. Our baby looked perfect to us.

When the procedure was over, the doctors and technician left the room and conferred. Then the ob-gyn came back in the room. "Well, it looks like we've got a mass," he told us. "Let me show it to you."

He pointed out a dark spot on the screen that the technician had measured but not described to us. It was, he told us, a tumor the size of a small grapefruit on my right ovary. Because it had grown quickly—there'd been no sign of it two and a half months earlier when I'd had a thorough ultrasound of the pelvic region—the doctors considered it very threatening. In fact, the doctor recommended surgery that day.

Steve and I were numb, then terrified. And we had many questions: Would a general anesthetic harm the baby? I'd given up my occasional glass of white wine and my morning cappuccino; surgery meant all types of drugs going through my veins. Still, the doctor assured us that a limited amount of anesthetic would not harm our baby's development. And he told us that if a woman must have surgery while pregnant, the fifth month was one of the best times. Earlier surgery carries a greater risk of miscarriage, and later surgery could trigger premature labor.

How would the doctor remove the tumor without disturbing the baby? He explained that he would make a vertical incision down the center of my stomach, gently move the baby aside and cut out the tumor.

I called my longtime gynecologist for a consultation, and I discussed the matter with my husband and parents. We all agreed that I had no other choice than to go ahead with the operation.

Four doctors were in the operating room for the procedure. The surgical team removed the tumor and, with it, my right ovary. The tissue was immediately sent to the lab for analysis.

When the results came back from the lab, one of the doctors left the operating room to give my family the diagnosis. "Well, the news is not good," he said. "The baby is fine and made it through the surgery very well, but the tumor we took out of Elisa was malignant. She has ovarian cancer."

They gave me the news when I woke up: "You have cancer." Those were the worst words I'd ever heard. As a reporter, I've interviewed so many desperate people in horrible situations that hearing I had cancer felt surreal, like a tragic news story that was happening to someone else.

Now there were serious decisions to make. If the cancer had spread and I needed radiation or chemotherapy, I might be able to carry the baby until seven months, the doctor said, when it would be able to live on its own, and then start treatment after I delivered. But if the cancer was aggressive, I might have to have chemotherapy right away. During surgery the medical team gathered a number of tissue samples from other organs, which were then sent to the lab for analysis to see if the cancer had spread. We would have to wait several days for those results.

A nurse hooked up a fetal monitor to my stomach, and I could hear my baby's quick heartbeat. It was like rhythmic music swirling in my head. I desperately hoped to continue carrying this baby.

Groggy from the pain medication, I fell asleep. When I awoke in the middle of the night, I saw Steve hunched over in a chair beside me, fast asleep. I felt so much love for him. We'd believed that with our infertility ordeal behind us, we were finally on our way to having a family. Now, during this one horrible day, he'd been told his wife had cancer and that his baby's life was in jeopardy. Still, he did his best to cheer and support me, and he stayed with me every night for the four nights I was in the hospital.

I talked a lot with Steve about my fears. When you hear you have cancer, all of a sudden you picture yourself bald from chemotherapy, skinny and frail, lying in a hospital bed. I kept telling myself that cancer is not necessarily a death sentence, and many people beat it. "It's just not my time to die yet," I told Steve. "I have so much more to do. Mostly, I just want to be a mother."

The next few days were the longest of my life. When my doctor appeared on his evening rounds on the third day, he announced the news we'd all prayed for: "Your cancer was confined to the right ovary. It was completely encapsulated.

"That means," he continued, "that when we removed the cancerous ovary, we took out every trace of the disease. You won't need any further treatment." He was 95 percent sure I was cured of the cancer, he said, and the odds don't get much better than that. Barring other complications, he said I should be able to deliver a healthy baby right on schedule.

Just as the joyful news started to sink in, my doctor told me something amazing.

"Your baby probably saved your life." He explained that I was only able to feel the abdominal pain that alerted us to the cancer because my growing uterus was pressing against the tumor. Had I not been pregnant, I might not have had any signs of the cancer until the tumor was very large and the disease much more advanced.

Ovarian cancer is one of the most deadly forms of the disease. According to the American Cancer Society, each year 26,700 women find out they have ovarian cancer, but only 44 percent of them live more than five years after the diagnosis. That's because it so often goes undetected: Usually there are no obvious symptoms until a woman's abdomen becomes enlarged, and at that point it's often too late. To catch the disease early, women need a thorough physical examination by a gynecologist and possibly an ultrasound of their reproductive organs to rule out any suspected problems. Even then, my doctor explained, catching the disease is a matter of luck. After all, my tumor hadn't been visible during my ultrasound ten weeks earlier.

Overwhelmed with relief, I smiled and wiped my eyes, hugging everyone in sight.

Later, when my family went to the hospital cafeteria to grab a bite, I walked alone to the maternity ward to see the brand-new babies. Up until then, I had avoided the place. I didn't want to see those tiny faces for fear I might never be able to deliver my baby there. Now, standing in my robe and slippers, I peered through the glass at the row of sleeping newborns. I stood with one hand on my stomach and wept.

I eventually returned to my job as a television reporter.

Viewers saw me get a little rounder each day. Soon the snow melted in the mountains, and daffodils started shooting up through the ground. I was ready to become a mother.

Four months after my surgery, I delivered a healthy nine-pound baby girl. We named her Mariel, which means "wished-for child." She has big, blue inquisitive eyes, and maybe someday she'll be a reporter like her mom.

I call Mariel my little angel. I know all mothers adore their infants, but how many can say, "I owe my life to my baby"?

Elisa Kayser Klein

A Gift of Love

There is no difficulty that enough love will not conquer.

Emmet Fox

Two years after an ectopic pregnancy and a bleak diagnosis for any chance of conceiving, my husband and I decided to adopt a baby. Always surrounded by family with children in abundance, we realized that it didn't matter how our baby arrived in this world. We just knew that our lives would not be complete without children to share the love we had to offer. Once the decision was made, we acted upon it immediately and registered with several adoption agencies. Unfortunately, the agencies offered little hope, and we knew in our hearts that our only real chance of adopting a baby would be through independent adoption.

We retained an adoption attorney and, following his advice, began placing ads in newspapers throughout the state. We set up a separate telephone line with an answering machine, then waited. At first, we had little response, but after a few weeks of consistent advertising, we began to receive calls. Our lawyer had given us a list of questions we could politely ask, which turned out to be extremely helpful since I was so nervous whenever the phone rang that I could barely remember my name, let alone ask anything meaningful. Throughout the next several months, I waded through obscene calls, pranksters and a few slim prospects, never getting over the heart palpitations and trembling that each phone call evoked. Eventually, I spoke with Julia.

Julia was four months pregnant, unwed, young and poor. She invited us to her house in a nearby town, and we gratefully accepted the invitation. As I walked up her rickety front steps, I remember taking a deep breath and thinking that my whole future depended on these next few moments. When she answered the door, I almost cried. She was so beautiful. Long, dirty-blonde hair framed her face, blue eyes sparkled with curiosity, and I could just make out the slightest rise in her stomach. We met both her mother and grandmother, and as three generations of women grilled us about our principles and beliefs, I silently prayed that we would be found worthy of their precious gift.

After three interminably long hours, we were hugged at the door as we departed. I was so elated on the trip home that I couldn't stop jabbering. "Did you see her tiny nose?" I asked my husband, who immediately laughed since our own rather large noses were almost literally a bone of contention. Over the next few months, with our attorney as mediator, we helped Julia with expenses related to her pregnancy. We paid for her doctor checkups and maternity clothes, and I had nightly conversations with Julia about her health and welfare. I felt as if she were my sister, feeling bonded in a way that was nurturing for both of us. Which was why it was so incredibly devastating when in her eighth month, Julia decided to keep her baby. The loss was as profound as my ectopic pregnancy had been; perhaps even worse because I was much further along in this pregnancy. I took to my bed for the next three days, barely able to eat, crying constantly, unwilling to speak with anyone but my husband. I was in mourning, and I desperately needed to grieve.

As difficult as it was, I continued to place ads, watching the months drag by with no response and little hope of my dream ever being fulfilled. It was two weeks after Christmas when my lawyer called me at work to ask if I could leave within the hour to go upstate and meet with a woman who had given birth to a baby two weeks before. Aurea was from the Philippines, unwed and visiting with family friends. She needed to go home, but there was no way she could take her baby with her. Being an unwed mother was a disgrace in her country, and she would be unable to provide for her child by herself. She had answered the ad of another couple who were clients of my lawyer and who, as Orthodox Jews, could not adopt a Filipino baby. Since Aurea had made the initial contact with my lawyer, it was completely legal for him to notify me of Aurea and her child. Within two hours, my husband and I had met shy, sweet Aurea and her beautiful baby boy. When she held him out to me, our eyes met, and I saw hope mingled with pain, the smile on her face only there to offer me support. I held him close, smelling his precious baby smell, not wanting to appear too aggressive, yet barely able to suppress my excitement. We stayed for an hour, communication shaky at best. When we left, it was agreed that Aurea would place her baby with us. She just needed a little more time to say good-bye to him.

The next week was a living nightmare. We searched our souls, desperately trying to confirm that we could handle loving and raising a racially different child. The loving part was no problem, but we weren't foolish enough to think that raising him would be simple. We didn't care. The adage, "love can conquer all," was to be our future motto. During the same week, Aurea had changed her mind. Not about us; she simply didn't want to part with her son, and who could blame her? I felt differently this time. I experienced no bitterness or anger. I understood.

But by the end of the week, she told my lawyer to have us come. It was snowing that day. A storm was predicted, but nothing would stop us. When we arrived, Aurea had dressed her baby in his finest clothes. She handed my husband a plastic bag filled with the articles she had acquired for her child over the past three weeks. She placed the baby in my arms and hugged me close, whispering in my ear, "Please, take care of my baby." "Always," I whispered back, sobbing as I left her crying in the kitchen and walked to my car. My husband, tears streaming down his face, backed out of the driveway. We headed home, all three of us, our hearts filled with love and gratitude, mingled with sorrow for Aurea's pain.

We never changed our son's first name. We felt it was the best gift we could give both him and Aurea. He is now twelve years old, and Aurea's act of kindness lives on daily in our hearts and souls.

Phyllis DeMarco

To My Child

Children are the purpose of life. We were once children and someone took care of us. Now it is our turn to care.

Cree Elder

I can feel you eagerly kick and move side to side. I cannot see you or even know your thoughts. When I go to sleep, walk around or when I wake you are there. You must wonder why this capsule you are in has so much turbulence. It must sound like a rainstorm to you when the beads of water from the shower are pounding on my belly.

I do know that you are aware of my emotions. When I am calm, you too seem calm. When I am crying or am terribly fatigued from stress, your kicks and ungraceful movements seem stronger than ever. It is as if you're saying, "Come on, Mom, hang in there, because if you don't, I can't."

To be very honest, I did not know that you were going to happen; you surprised me. However, you are a very loved and accepted person by me, and many other people. I guess you are used to my voice by now. They tell me that you can hear things in your little gestation cap-sule. Can you? You haven't heard your father's voice. Do you wonder why? Just know that he also loves you.

When I awoke this morning I lay there with my tummy bare and watched you push my stomach up with your feet. I wish I could have shared this unforgettable experi-ence with someone. God was smiling down at you; remember he creates no accidents. My desire to have con-ceived you in the right marriage situation is very strong, yet that makes you no less of a person, nor does it take from the incredible love and bond I have with you.

I apologize if some of the foods I eat for both of us aren't what you like. If I knew what your favorite food was, I swear that I would eat it. Oh yes, and my music: I know you must hear it. I love music as I'm sure you already are aware. Are you a Bing Crosby fan or are you a rhythm-and-blues baby?

I know that after you are born and I hold you and nurse you, I will be even more in love. When I see that you resemble myself, my parents or even your father, that bond will be intensified. That is why when I hand you to your new parents, it will without a doubt be the most dif-ficult and painful thing I'll ever have to do. I know that in my head and in God's eyes it is the right thing to do for you. If I kept you for my own it would be selfish. Everything I do, I am doing because I love you with all my heart.

I will always be your birth mother and you will always be my biological child, although I may never see you again. And if I did, I would never reject you. I love you.

Heather James

How Bubba Lukey Got His Name

We named our first son Sam. We loved him so much we decided to have another. When my wife, Leah, got into the second trimester, we started talking about names. We both wanted something biblical, but that was where the agreement ended.

One evening after dinner I ran a few possibilities by her. "How about Moses?" I asked, half seriously. "We could call him 'Moe' for short."

Leah didn't go for that.

"What about Nimrod?" I asked. "Nimrod the mighty hunter."

She just rolled her eyes and turned away. But later, she pitched a few names of her own: "Jacob?"

Nope. Too popular.

"Matthew?"

Nope. We almost named our first son Matthew. I couldn't dish out a leftover to our new son.

Then one day, sitting together at a Bible study, we came across the name Simeon: ". . . when she gave birth to a son . . . she named him Simeon" (Gen. 29:33). The "she" in the passage is Leah, and as the story goes, Simeon was Leah's second son. There was a kind of neat symmetry about the whole thing.

"Hey," I said, nudging Leah, "what about Simeon?"

"What about Simon?"

Close enough. We had ourselves a name, or so I thought. A few days later my wife came and said, "Ix-nay on Simon."

"Why?" I asked. "What's wrong with Simon?"

"People will make fun of his name. They'll call him Simple Simon."

"But what about the biblical second-son-of-Leah thing?" I asked.

"Here's the deal," said my wife. "We name him Simon, but we call him something else. Simon doesn't have to be a first name. It can be his middle name."

So it was back to the name books. We tried Aaron and Zack, Jack and Shaq, Moby and Toby. None of them stuck.

Meanwhile, my wife's belly grew rounder. One fall Saturday afternoon while I was watching football, she came to me and said, "Hey, how about Luke?"

"Luke." I said it aloud. I repeated it a few times. It sounded good.

"And the best part," she said, "is that no one can make fun of it."

"It's insult-proof," I said. "Luke Simon Doughty."

So we were agreed.

Until Sunday, at least. I was watching another football game when my wife came in and said, "It won't work."

I knew at once what she was referring to. "What's wrong now?"

"His monogram: Luke Simon Doughty equals LSD. I can't have my son's initials be a major hallucinogen."

"Look," I said, turning off the football game. "It's a bit late to be fooling with names again, don't you think?"

My wife stood there shaking her head. "I can't do it. My son will not have the initials LSD."

Then I had the answer. "What if we name him Simon Luke Doughty, but call him by his middle name?"

She thought for a moment, then nodded. "Yes, Simon Luke Doughty, but we'll call him Luke. Works for me."

Relieved, I went back to my game.

The very next Thursday, Leah delivered our baby boy— a cheeky seven-pounder, a delight just like his brother. On Saturday, we brought Baby Luke home, and family and friends came by with gifts and covered casseroles, hoping to catch a glimpse of the new bubba. Big brother Sam was as excited as anyone. "Can I hold Baby Wookey?" he asked all evening.

When things had settled down, I took Sam upstairs for bedtime. We knelt to pray beside his bed, and Sam added the "God blesses": "God bless Mama and Daddy, God bless Sammy and"—and why didn't I see this coming?— "and God bless Luke the Kook."

Del Doughty

The Mouth That Roared

I couldn't wait for my son to talk. Those first golden words, that first raggedy sentence: "More eat, Mom!"

Only later did I realize how little control I had over what he'd say—and when he'd say it. Shortly after Sam turned three, a new security guard appeared at day care. He was an older man with thinning hair; to compensate, he'd combed the few remaining strands jaggedly across his scalp. Not that I noticed until Sam called it to my attention.

"Mom, look! That man has broken hair!" I froze. Sam repeated himself, louder. "Hey, mister—you've got broken hair!" As the man's entire head turned red, I winced, gave a "kids say the darndest things" shrug by way of apology, and hustled Mr. Observant into the car.

It was as good a place as any to start teaching him diplomacy. "I think you hurt that man's feelings," I said gently. "He knows he doesn't have much hair." I stopped for a light and checked the rearview mirror to see if I was getting through. Sam stared back blankly. "Okay," I continued. "What if someone said, 'Wow! What funny-looking teeth!' That would bother you, right?"

Silence from the back. And then . . .

"Mom?"

"Yes, honey?"

"You have funny teeth!" he crowed, and giggled all the way home.

I began to see what I might be up against. And no wonder: Hadn't we encouraged Sam to notice the world around him? "See the pretty kitty!" "Look at that big moon!" And hadn't we bragged about Sam's own candid assessments? A few weeks before the broken-hair incident, at an Italian restaurant, we ordered that child-friendly staple, mozzarella sticks. Sam nibbled one and pushed away the plate. A waiter later came by and asked Sam if he liked his entreé, spaghetti. "Yes," he said, then pointed to his neglected appetizer. "But those are terrible!"

For weeks we laughed about Sam, Kid Critic: Yes, the mozzarella sticks were terrible! What a great little palate!

He was spontaneous, bright, open—everything we cherish in children. Only now did I see how it had led us to a balding man's humiliation. We'd taught our son to be observant; what we hadn't shown him was when and why to keep his observations to himself.

And so we tread warily in public with Sam, a walking, talking time bomb. What would set him off next? One day, he hailed a couple of elderly women. "You'd like my grandmother," he assured them. "She's old, too." Another time he waved away a smoker: "Hey, you're going to die!"

Each time, we'd stammer an apology and sweep Sam off for a chat. We'd explain that no, we don't tell people they're old or that smoking will kill them. It may be true, but for us to say so would only make them feel bad. We eventually boiled it down to "If you can't say something nice, don't say anything at all." Unfortunately, "nice" proved a relative term.

We found that out just after Sam's fourth birthday, when my husband invited an old friend to dinner—a genial, portly man whose girth Sam obviously found mesmerizing. Despite our attempts at diversion, Sam stared until he could stand it no longer. Finally, he stepped right up and tapped the man on the belly. "Boy," he said, with genuine admiration, "you're fat!"

I stared into my wine, wishing I could drown in it, as our (childless) guest valiantly tried to laugh it off. It wasn't until dessert that we regained our equilibrium.

The next day, we had another sedan sermonette. "We do not tell people they're fat, old or bald," I said. This time, when I peeked into the rearview mirror, I saw a gleam of comprehension. It dawned on me that the four-year-old was grappling with a notion the three-year-old couldn't have fathomed: that words could embarrass or hurt. "Sorry," Sam said, squirming.

Just how far Sam had come became clear weeks later, when I took him to my health club for a swim. As we passed the stair-climbing machines, an acquaintance caught my eye. He was a friendly, good-looking man whose left arm ended just below the shoulder. I smiled, or tried to, gritting my teeth as I imagined what Sam might say. As I pulled him along, his eyes widened, but he said nothing.

The next day, I complimented Sam on his restraint.

"Remember the man we saw at the health club, who had only one arm?" Sam, busy dismantling a Lego dinosaur, nodded.

"I'm very proud of you. You noticed something was different, but you didn't say anything. That's great!"

"He knows he has one arm, Mom," he replied, patiently. "I didn't want to hurt his feelings."

"That's right." By God, he had it! And then . . .

"Mom? Could we take his picture?"

Maybe we have more work to do.

Barbara Hoffman

Tears

Tears are the safety valve of the heart when too much pressure is laid on.

Albert Smith

"I can't find a heartbeat." Dr. Deasy said these words with no evidence of emotion. His graying hair was a bit tousled, but he was completely professional as he glided his Doppler scope over my glistening (and already swelling) abdomen. He adjusted his glasses, as if seeing more clearly could somehow help him to hear a beating heart more distinctly. I began to feel just a little nervous but was not yet overly apprehensive. Surely he had just not found the right spot yet. If he kept trying, he'd find the baby's heartbeat. I knew that a baby was sometimes in a position that made it awkward for the Doppler to pick up the sound of its beating heart.

"You are a little larger than you should be at fourteen weeks. There is a possibility that you have a placenta growing at an abnormal rate, but no actual fetus inside."

"What?"

"It could be a 'false' pregnancy. Or, it is possible that

you were pregnant, but the child did not survive. In that case, your body may have reacted by overproducing the hormones necessary to sustain a pregnancy, creating the appearance of a more advanced state of pregnancy."

Now I was definitely apprehensive. My husband, standing beside me, squeezed my hand. All of the old feelings came back. Three times before, I had lost babies to miscarriage early in pregnancy. Three times, I had mourned the loss of little ones I would never know. But the intensity of that grief had been eased when I successfully carried two babies to full term.

I don't think that those we love are ever "replaced" by someone else. Still, as we move toward other relationships, the pain of loss is lessened. My two healthy baby boys (now toddlers of one and two) had given me so much joy that the ache over my earlier losses had been overcome, if not forgotten. And certainly my "successful" pregnancies had given me confidence that the old problems were in the past.

Now here I was, faced with the old feelings again. How quickly those tears rose to the surface! For someone who has never experienced miscarriage, it may be hard to relate to the ordeal I was facing. I know that many of my friends did not understand it at the time. I would never presume that the anguish I experienced was even close to that of a mother who loses a child she has grown to know and love. I doubt seriously that anything could equal that torment. But there is a unique connection that develops between mother and child long before they ever meet face to face. Love begins to grow as a mother becomes increasingly aware of the tiny life within her. When that life is abruptly cut off, the grief experienced is as real as that for any other loss.

I left the doctor's office that day in stunned disbelief. I had an appointment to get an ultrasound that afternoon, but there were several hours to wait. Since the doctor's office was closer to my mom's house than it was to ours, we went over there to wait the long hours before we could get into the hospital for an ultrasound—and confirmation of our loss. My parents were out of town, but I had a key, so we let ourselves in. As I sat on the bed making phone calls, the tears began to flow. I called my aunt and my pastor's wife to ask for prayer. They comforted me, assured me of their love and prayers, and promised to call a few others to pray as we waited. Steve held me, and we both held the boys, gaining comfort and strength from one another.

As the hours of waiting passed slowly, I allowed myself to slip into depression. All the confidence of my two successful pregnancies disappeared. I managed to brace myself against the loss I was facing by putting up walls against the pain. When I walked into the hospital that afternoon, I was emotionally prepared for the worst. I had cried all my tears and was ready to accept the news I most feared. A knot had formed in the pit of my stomach from the stress I had dumped there. I knew that I may have gained control over my emotions, but my body would continue to feel the pain, refusing to be subdued by my tears.

Since we had the two boys with us, Steve was unable to come into the room with me as I received my ultrasound. I got up onto the cold, hard table and waited for the technician to begin. She was friendly and supportive, but somewhat "businesslike" in her efficiency, as she began the procedure. As a technician, she was not legally allowed to give me any diagnosis, but it was not long before it was easy to read her demeanor. She changed from having a guarded, professional approach to a relaxed and positive attitude. Although she couldn't make a diagnosis, she could let me see the screen as she glided the ultrasonic head over my abdomen. She did not have to say a word.

There, on the screen in front of me, I clearly saw the active and very much alive movements of the small child inside me. I could even see this tiny creature (only fourteen weeks since the day of conception) sucking its tiny thumb as it floated freely around the amniotic fluid in my body.

I was flooded with relief. I don't think I knew until that instant just how much I had truly feared the loss of this child. Now the tears, which I had thought were under control, began to flow again. This time they were tears of joy and comfort. At that moment I did not think that anything could make me happier than the joy of having a healthy child inside me. But I was wrong.

When the technician had finished her job, she went out of the room to make her report to the radiologist. I had to wait to hear the good news officially from him. When he walked into the room, he asked me how I was. "Fine," I said. "Terrific, in fact, now that I've seen the baby."

"Which baby did you see?"

I thought it was a rather silly question.

"Mine, of course."

"But which one did you see?"

"Huh? What do you mean? I saw the one inside me now."

He was grinning, as if he were in on some sort of conspiracy. "But, there are two in there. Didn't you notice? You are pregnant with twins!"

No. I hadn't noticed. It hadn't even occurred to me that the technician had been wandering all over my tummy with that ultrasound head and showing me first one baby and then another; I had been so excited and relieved to see a living, moving baby, that I hadn't noticed. She had never shown them both at once, and I just assumed it was the same baby.

Steve, waiting patiently and prayerfully out in the hall with the boys, was now asked to come into the room. The radiologist then showed us both babies on the screen, as we watched in amazement.

The ride home from the hospital was a dramatic contrast to the ride we had taken earlier that same day from the doctor's office to my parents' house. Once again, we were stunned and having a hard time grasping the news. But our grief and fear had been swept away and emphatically replaced by joy and hope. There were still long moments of silence, but they were underscored now by laughter, amazement and wonder. Admittedly, there was a new sort of apprehension in me. I was facing an entirely new and unforeseen challenge. But the only tears now were tears of joy.

Bonnie J. Mansell

Miracle Baby

Hope is putting faith to work when doubting would be easier.

E. C. McKenzie

When Sara Sieber was sixteen weeks pregnant, she and her husband, Tim, went to her obstetrician's office for a routine ultrasound. The couple was looking forward to finding out whether their baby would be a boy or a girl. The sonogram showed that Sara was carrying a son, her fourth. But there was no time to celebrate the happy news, because the scan also revealed a serious defect.

Sara's baby's diaphragm, the thin wall of muscle and connective tissue that separates the abdomen from the chest, was not forming properly. The condition is known as congenital diaphragmatic hernia. Minor cases can usually be repaired surgically shortly after birth. But the entire left half of Sara's baby's diaphragm was missing. His tiny stomach and liver were pushing their way into his chest cavity, leaving his tissue-thin lungs with absolutely no room to grow.

"Your baby has virtually no lungs at all," the neonatologist explained as he reviewed a second, more detailed set of ultrasounds. "I'm afraid there's no hope. I would strongly recommend that you terminate the pregnancy immediately."

"I can't do that!" Sara gasped, clutching Tim's hand in a white-knuckled grip.

"If you carry your baby to term, he will almost certainly suffocate to death at birth," the neonatologist said sadly. "There's a small chance we could keep him alive for up to several months on a ventilator, but then he would die anyway."

"I felt like the whole world had dropped out from under me," recalls Sara. "I'd suffered two previous miscarriages, but they'd happened early in my pregnancies. This was different. I could feel this baby moving inside me. I was already in love with him, and now the doctor was telling me I would never get to hold him in my arms."

As Sara and Tim stood to leave, both of them in tears, the doctor remembered something he'd read in a recent medical journal. "There's a surgeon in California who's trying to operate on babies with this condition while they're still in the womb. It's highly experimental, and I don't believe he's had much success, but I can make a few calls, at least."

Sara wasn't hopeful. "By the time we got home, I was already grieving the loss of my baby," she says. "I didn't want him to be born, because as soon as he was born I knew I was going to lose him."

Four days later, the doctor telephoned with a name: Dr. Michael Harrison with the Fetal Treatment Center at the University of California at San Francisco. Sara and Tim decided they had little to lose, so in February of 1996, the couple flew from North Carolina to California for an evaluation.

As babies develop inside the uterus, fluid forms in their lungs and flows out their mouths, contributing to the amniotic fluid that cushions and protects the growing fetus. Dr. Harrison proposed to use this very fluid to help Sara's baby's lungs grow bigger. The surgeon would temporarily close off the baby's trachea. The fluid would then build up inside his lungs, and the mounting pressure would cause them to expand like inflated balloons.

During the previous two and a half years, Dr. Harrison had attempted the procedure on eleven babies. Only one had survived. But in ten of these cases, Harrison had opened the mother's uterus to operate on the fetus, which usually precipitated a preterm delivery before the babies' lungs had any time to grow.

More recently, Harrison had devised newer, less invasive techniques. Instead of cutting open the mother's uterus, Harrison was now prepared to perform the surgery orthoscopically. So far he'd tried the improved techniques on only one baby, which had subsequently died.

"You're an excellent candidate for the surgery, but I'm not going to give you any false hopes," Harrison told the Siebers.

During their visit Sara and Tim also consulted with a hospital obstetrician and a social worker. Both strongly advised the couple not to proceed.

"We've seen what these mothers go through, both emotionally and physically, and their babies die, anyway," the obstetrician argued.

The social worker reminded Sara that she had three children back home: Timmy, now nine, Ryan, seven and Jacob, four. "You'd have to move to San Francisco for at least six months. Imagine how that long an absence might affect them."

During the flight home, Sara made up her mind. "I'm not going back there," she told Tim. From the start, Tim's primary concern had been his wife's health. But thus far all of the mothers had come through the surgery without serious complications. "This is the only chance we have to help our baby live," he reminded Sara. "Maybe we should give this more thought, discuss it with our doctor back home."

There wasn't much time. Sara was already twenty-four weeks pregnant. For the surgery to succeed it had to be done by week thirty, because after that the baby's lungs would begin to produce increasingly less of the vital fluid.

Sara and Tim prayed over their decision. They consulted their obstetrician, who told them, "I've seen too many babies choke to death because they simply don't have enough lungs to draw their first breath. If there's anything you can do, no matter how slim the chances . . ."

The Siebers's minister agreed. "You've been given the knowledge that this surgery exists. You have to do whatever you can, and then trust in God to do the rest."

"I still wasn't any more hopeful," Sara remembers. "But I thought, maybe the doctor could learn something that might eventually help some other baby to survive."

The couple left their three sons with Tim's parents, and before they returned to California, they named their unborn child Samuel. "We named him in honor of the Bible story of Hannah, who dedicated her son's life to God," says Sara.

Dr. Harrison began the four-hour operation by making a transverse C-section incision in Sara's abdomen. A sonographer then helped him gently maneuver the baby face-up inside the womb and suture a single stitch through his chin to hold his neck in place.

Next, Harrison made three pencil-thin holes in Sara's uterus and amniotic sack with surgical trocars—hollow tubes through which he manipulated his instruments, a saline pump to keep the amniotic fluid clear and a camera to monitor his every move. With slow precision the surgeon guided a pair of long-handled orthoscopic scissors toward the baby's neck and snipped a single, small cut.

He parted the skin, and then used a special, titanium lip to close off the baby's trachea.

"That should do it," Harrison announced to his team as he prepared to close. The operation had gone remarkably well, and the surgeon felt cautiously optimistic.

Dr. Harrison hoped that Samuel would remain inside his mother's womb until he reached his thirty-fifth week—five weeks shy of full term. But the moment Sara came out of the anesthesia she felt sticky and wet.

"What's wrong?" she groggily asked a nurse.

"Your water just broke," the nurse replied, and hurried off to find the doctor. Despite Dr. Harrison's best efforts, the trauma of surgery had taken its toll. Sara's sack had ruptured, and preterm labor was imminent. Yet it wasn't uncommon for a twenty-eight-and-a-half-week preemie to survive with the aid of warming beds and respirators. But not Samuel. With no time for the trachea clip to do its job, Sara's baby seemed fated to die.

But then something remarkable happened. Somehow, the baby shifted position inside the sack, and his tiny head stanched the leak. Slowly, the amniotic fluid began to replenish itself. The pressure inside Samuel's lungs also continued to rise, and within a few days sonograms revealed substantial lung growth.

"God had intervened, and I was convinced everything was going to be fine," says Sara. But on the twelfth day post-surgery, a second complication arose.

The morning Sara was scheduled to be released from the hospital to a nearby Ronald McDonald House she developed a painful infection that put both her life and the baby's at risk. This time there could be no reprieve. Live or die—Samuel had to be born.

Dr. Harrison performed a partial C-section, delivering only the baby's head and neck. He removed the titanium clip and sutured shut the skin. He put in a breathing tube connected to a high-frequency respirator that delivered over three hundred gentle puffs of air every minute. Only then did the surgeon complete the delivery and cut the umbilical cord.

Samuel was nine weeks premature, and weighed a mere three pounds, nine and a half ounces. "He made it this far. That's got to be a good sign," Dr. Harrison insisted, but other members of the neonatal ICU staff weren't nearly so hopeful.

"You need to prepare yourself. He's not going to live," more than one doctor told the Siebers bluntly.

"They kept Samuel so heavily sedated, for the first two weeks of his life I really couldn't tell if he was alive," recalls Sara. "We prayed and prayed, but no matter what happened, Tim and I both agreed we'd made the right decision to try."

Hour by hour, day by day, little Samuel defied the odds and clung tenaciously to life. When he was a week old Dr. Harrison performed surgery to install a Gore-Tex patch to replace the missing left half of his diaphragm. Two more operations would follow—the first to repair a bilateral hernia and a second to correct a bowel obstruction.

When Samuel was five weeks old, Sara finally got to hold him in her arms for the very first time. "His skin was so translucent, I could trace the map of blood vessels across his tiny body," she says. "I told him how much I loved him, and all about his three brothers who couldn't wait for us to bring him home."

Even at two and a half months, Sara was still being told by the NICU doctors, "Don't get your hopes up. He's still not out of the woods." But Samuel's lungs continued to develop and grow stronger.

Then, late one evening, Sara and Tim received a phone call at their hotel room. "You might want to come back to the hospital," a nurse told them. "We've removed the breathing tube. Samuel is breathing on his own."

"His feeble cries sounded like a tiny, lost kitten," Sara vividly recalls. "After twelve long weeks of prayer and worry, I couldn't imagine a sweeter sound."

Two weeks later, Samuel was strong enough to fly home to North Carolina. Members of the Siebers's church met them at the airport carrying a large sign: "Welcome home, Samuel! We love you!" Fellow passengers who had heard the story applauded and cheered as Sara deplaned with her precious cargo cradled snugly in her arms.

That was in July of 1996. Today, more than two years later, Sara's youngest has grown into a happy, active child who loves riding his tricycle and playing on the backyard swing set with his three brothers.

Samuel's right lung has reached normal size for his age, though his left lung is only about one-fourth of the normal size. "The Gore-Tex patch will need to be replaced as he grows older, but he hasn't had a lot of problems they thought he might have," says Tim Sieber.

"We're all very pleased with how well Samuel has done," says Dr. Harrison. "He's been a true inspiration for our ongoing work." Indeed, since Samuel's birth, Harrison and his team have used their refined surgical techniques to operate on eleven more infants with congenital diaphragmatic hernias, and eight are alive and doing well.

One who was particularly moved by Samuel's success was the hospital social worker who had originally tried to talk Sara out of undergoing the surgery. "The day before I got to take Samuel home she came by and asked if she could hold him," Sara relates. "There were tears in her eyes, and she kept saying again and again, 'You're nothing but a miracle. You're nothing but a miracle.'"

Bill Holton

Lesson in Courage

Birth is the sudden opening of a window through which you look out upon a stupendous prospect.

William Dixon

Numbly, I walked through the neonatal intensive care unit.

"He's been through so much," I breathed, as I peered at my little boy in his incubator. How long can he keep going like this?

"He's a fighter," doctors had told me. But in my heart, I couldn't find the courage to hope. Little did I imagine it would be this little fighter himself who would teach me the meaning of courage. . . .

My husband Jon and I had rejoiced when we found ourselves staring at a positive home pregnancy test.

"A baby brudder—or sister!" cried Samantha, four, and Emma, three.

Then one night when I was just twenty-four weeks along, a sharp pain and a gush of fluid jarred me awake. "Something's wrong," I panicked.

"There's a small tear in your amniotic sac," the doctor

said. He hoped medication would delay my labor until the baby's lungs could develop. But one week later, contractions started.

"You have a uterine infection," the doctor said. "We have to deliver the baby now, or we could lose you both!"

"No!" I sobbed. "It's too soon!"

Holding me, Jon soothed, "Everything's going to be okay. He's going to be a fighter, just like you. You'll see."

But inside, I knew he was wrong about my being a fighter, because with each contraction, fear tore through me. *How can I bear to lose this baby?* I anguished.

Seven hours later, Sean Eric Fox, weighing just one pound, seven ounces, came into the world without so much as a peep and was whisked to intensive care before I could hold him.

The next day, when I saw him for the first time, I was filled with despair. Unlike the healthy, pink babies his sisters had been, Sean had lobster-red skin. His eyes were closed. And he had so many tubes, I couldn't find a place on his body to touch.

"Is he going to make it?" I stammered.

"We're doing our best," his doctor answered. He explained that because Sean was so premature, his lungs so underdeveloped, there was a chance of blindness, brain damage, death. "A lot will depend on Sean," he added. "If he's a fighter, there's a chance."

But I barely heard his words.

"We're going to lose him!" I wept.

"No!" Jon insisted. "He's going to make it!"

Back home, I tried to carry on as if everything was okay. "When is Sean coming home?" the girls asked.

How could I explain that their little brother might *never* come home. Sitting by Sean's incubator, my heart pounded each time a monitor went off to signal his oxygen level had dropped. *What if they can't help him?* I'd panic as nurses rushed over.

And when, at three weeks, nurses finally let me hold Sean, I was so scared of hurting him. Yet as scared as I was, Sean seemed utterly fearless. Even when his lungs were working so poorly that his fingernails turned blue, he'd curl his hands into a tiny fist and swing them furiously as if to say, "I'm *not* giving up!"

I'm so proud of him, I often thought. But deep down, I worried how long he could keep fighting. Would I ever see him again? I wept when doctors said he needed surgery to repair a hernia that was strangling his intestines.

Though he came through the operation with flying colors, my heart ached with worry. And when his oxygen level dropped again, as it had so many times before, I couldn't hold back my tears. "He's not getting better," I wept. "He's never going to come home." But that evening as I sat in the intensive care unit watching Sean kick with all his might as the nurse changed his dressings, I couldn't help but smile. "I guess he really is a fighter," I chuckled.

"That's why he's come so far," the nurse said. "Whatever life throws his way, he fights back with everything he's got. That's why babies like Sean make it."

Hearing her words, a little twinge stabbed my heart. *She's right!* I gulped. No matter how many times his oxygen level dropped, no matter how high his fever raged, no matter how much pain he was in, Sean never gave up. Oh, I knew the doctors and nurses had fought hard to keep him alive, but I sensed there was something more keeping Sean going. *He doesn't know the odds are against him!* I realized. *All he knows is that he's alive and he's got to keep fighting—kicking those legs, churning those arms, clutching with those tiny fingers.*

If a six-week-old preemie can fight that hard, why can't I? I thought, brushing away a tear. *Constantly thinking about the worst that can happen isn't going to help anybody—not Sean, not my family, not me.* And though I wasn't sure how, I knew that, somehow, I had to be more like Sean.

"It's not going to be easy for an old worrier like your

mom to change her ways," I whispered. "But I promise, Sean, if you'll keep fighting, I'll try, too."

As if he understood every word, Sean squeezed my finger with all his might.

Until then, I'd been too afraid of hurting Sean to learn how to give him the special care he needed. Now, I reasoned, *the more I learned, the less scary it would be.* "Could you show me how his monitors work?" I asked his nurse.

At home the next day, when I peeked into the empty nursery, instead of feeling sorry for myself, I told myself to imagine Sean in my arms as I rocked him.

When the girls asked, "When is Sean coming home?" instead of sinking into despair, I'd say, "He's getting bigger every day—he gained a whole gram yesterday!"

A few weeks later, when I brought Samantha and Emma to see their baby brother for the first time, my heart filled with joy as they cooed in awe. To my amazement, I no longer doubted that Sean would one day climb the jungle gym in our yard with his big sisters. Slowly, I'd let hope fill my heart, and to my amazement, I'd discovered a strength I'd never known.

And as if Sean sensed my renewed spirit, he seemed to fight even harder. And after twelve weeks, he finally came home weighing a hefty three pounds, fourteen ounces!

"I told you he was a fighter!" Jon said as I took Sean to his own nursery for the first time. "Just like his mommy!"

"Thanks," I smiled. "But I learned everything I know about being a fighter from my son."

Today, Sean is a healthy toddler who loves Popsicles and playing peek-a-boo with his sisters. I'll always be inspired by the fighting spirit that saw him through those first hard days—and taught me everything I know about courage and hope.

Ami Fox as told to Dianne Gill
Excerpted from Woman's World

Dads Will Be Dads

While I was pregnant with my first child, sweltering through the endless, fiery summer months in which ankles swelled and sweat poured forth profusely, I wanted only one thing—to give birth.

"I can't wait until this child is out," I would huff and puff in frustration.

My husband lovingly reassured me that the baby would spring forth at the appointed time. That some day I would be free from the burden of the added weight and the painful swollen ankles. I, however, felt as if the child had taken up permanent residence.

"Suppose the kid likes it in here and doesn't want to leave," I would say.

"Highly unlikely, dear. The baby will be here before you know it," he insisted, his feet still grounded firmly in reality, while mine were constantly elevated.

As it turned out, when my water broke that fateful evening, I was shocked into reality. Our first daughter did leave the womb and enter the atmosphere. She even arrived three weeks early.

When Mary was born, I was overjoyed. Not only was it a relief to hold her tiny body in my arms, but she was a red-headed beauty. Even when she was minutes old, I felt that we had a unique attachment. And we did, for she had been a part of me. However, what I didn't anticipate was how difficult it would be to let her go.

For those nine months that seemed like an eternity, the baby had been mine . . . all mine. She was joined with me and depended on only me for survival. Even though Tom could feel her kick through the womb as she grew bigger, I usually had to notify him that she was moving. He depended on me to tell him what the baby was doing. The communication that Mary and I had was ours alone. Now, she was in the world and I had to share her with others. Including her dad.

Now, it's not that I didn't trust him. My husband is a compassionate husband and father. It's just that he doesn't do things the way that I do them.

He held the baby differently. I cradled her close, showing her my maternal love. He held her facing outward so she would have a world view. He transported her differently. I carried her in my arms from room to room as I tidied up. He placed her in the stroller and rolled her around so that he could put things away and still keep an eye on her. He comforted her differently. I rocked her quietly to calm her; he bounced her. He even fed her differently. I breast-fed her at 2:00 A.M. He bottle-fed her at 2:00 P.M. (Okay, so I can't hold biology against the poor guy.) It's just that it was difficult to accept that someone could relate to Mary in another way. Undoubtedly, I was very insecure, and sharing her was hard. Even with her dad.

Of course, there was the time that I was downstairs in the basement office for a while working on a project. It was Dad's time to watch his little girl. As I reached the top of the steps after finishing my work, he asked, "Where's Mary?"

"What do you mean, where is Mary?" I screamed.

"I thought you had her," he said nonchalantly. "Don't worry, I'll find her." He had placed her on the living-room floor for a moment and then inadvertently turned his back. We began our search there. As it turned out, she had crawled over to the floor-length picture window and was hiding behind the drapes. We found her giggling in delight at the birds on the front lawn and at the cars passing by. It was the first time that she had crawled. I seldom placed her on the floor, but Tom liked to give her room to stretch and play. No harm was done, in fact just the opposite. Our baby had reached a new point in her life because my husband, her dad, had let her expand her horizons.

During all those months of pregnancy while I complained, I never imagined how difficult it would be to let her go once she was born. For me, it was the first test of motherhood—to let Dad be Dad. To realize that someone else could nurture my child in his own way. And to realize that what he had to give her, I couldn't give.

That is the beauty of parenting. That each mother and each father has a unique contribution. That our babies need the distinctive love and nurture that each one of us has to offer. And it pays off, too. By the time our second child was on the way, Mary was two years old. She and her dad had a wonderful relationship forged by the variety of experiences which they alone had shared.

After our youngest child, Kristi, arrived, I was able to give my husband more freedom—and space—in his distinctive parenting techniques. I, too, had grown. And, I had learned from his parenting style, even as he had learned from mine. After all, we were a team.

"Well, they're all yours," I declared one day as I headed for the office.

"Aren't you just a little worried?" he teased.

"No, just remember to check behind the drapes if the baby disappears," I laughed. "Besides," I added, "you've got everything under control."

Susan M. Lang

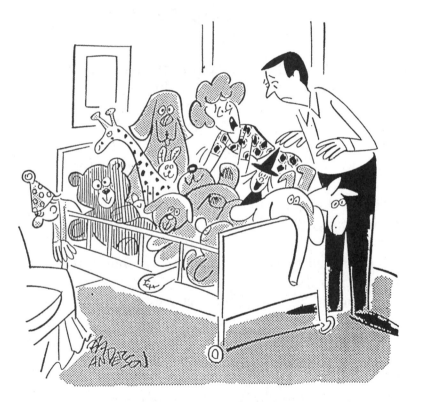

"Are you SURE you put her to bed?"

Reprinted by permission of George Crenshaw.

A Life or Death Decision

Amber Brittingham stood in the nursery doorway, tears streaming down her cheeks. Inside, her mom sat in the old wooden rocker singing "Jesus Loves You" and rocking Amber's infant daughter, Rachel, to sleep. *That should be me sitting there singing to my baby,* Amber thought miserably. But Amber was under strict doctor's orders not to touch her own baby, or even to stand too close.

Amber was grateful for all her mom's help, but Rachel was her baby, after all. *I don't want to watch Rachel from a distance,* she silently sobbed. "I want to feed her and put her to bed and all those other things I've waited my whole lifetime to do."

Ever since she was a little girl, Amber had dreamed of the day when she would start a family of her own. She could barely contain her joy when she learned she and her husband, Jonathan, were expecting their first child. But Amber's joy soon turned to sorrow and despair.

During a routine checkup at the beginning of her fourth month, Amber's doctor discovered a lima bean-size lump in her thyroid gland. A surgeon did a biopsy, and he called Saturday afternoon with the results.

Amber and Jonathan had planned to go out that night to celebrate her twenty-seventh birthday. Instead she called her mom. "I have thyroid cancer," she wept. "I don't know what I'm going to do."

Anne and Bob Marchant drove sixteen hours from Oklahoma, to Colorado Springs where Jonathan was stationed with the army. Monday morning they accompanied their daughter and son-in-law to the doctor's office. They all listened intently as the surgeon assured Amber, "Your prognosis is excellent. But we'll have to schedule the surgery as soon as possible."

Amber had a single question for the doctor. "How will the operation affect the baby?"

"It could cause premature labor," the surgeon allowed. "We might not be able to stop it."

Amber touched her swelling belly. The baby was only four-and-a-half months along. If it were born now, she knew it could never survive. "I have to wait," she instantly decided. "I can't risk hurting the baby."

Jonathan supported her decision, but Amber's folks wanted her to have the operation right away. "You're our baby. We only want what's best for you," they pleaded.

"I may be your baby, but please understand that right now this is my baby I'm fighting for," Amber replied. The doctor warned that if she waited, there was a chance the cancer could spread into her lymph nodes. But Amber's mind was set. "If I hadn't gotten pregnant I might never have discovered the cancer in time. This baby saved my life, and now I'm going to do whatever it takes to save its life."

Amber left the doctor's office convinced she'd made the right decision. "I can do this," Amber told her family and the other women at the preschool where she worked as a teacher. But every morning Amber woke up clutching her husband, all but paralyzed with fear. "Is the cancer spreading?" she worried. "Am I going to live or die?"

One day during her sixth month, Amber was driving home from work when the baby started kicking. Amber put a hand on her belly, and suddenly she could not hold back her tears. "What if I don't make it and somebody else has to raise my child?" she panicked. "What if I'm not there to tuck her in at night, or help her get dressed for her very first day of school?"

During her eighth month, doctors did an ultrasound on Amber's thyroid. Now, instead of a single cancerous nodule there were five. The cancer was growing, but Amber was determined to hold out for one last month. "Whatever happens to me, at least the baby will make it," she comforted herself.

On Amber's due date doctors induced labor and delivered a healthy baby girl. "I did it," Amber rejoiced, counting fingers and toes. "Look," she told Jonathan, "our baby is perfect."

Amber took her baby home, but she had little time to enjoy being a new mom. It was time for Amber to begin her cancer treatment—and pray to God it wasn't too late.

Amber's parents and husband paced the waiting room as a two-hour thyroidectomy stretched into five. "The cancer was even worse than we thought," the surgeon explained when Amber awoke in the recovery room. The cancer had spread dangerously close to Amber's vocal cords, and now she couldn't say a word. "There's a chance the damage to your vocal cords may be permanent," the doctor grimly reported.

Amber's mom took time off work to care for Rachel while her daughter convalesced. But the surgery had left Amber so weak, she could barely get out of bed. When Anne brought the baby in, Amber didn't have the strength to hold her, or the voice to say "I love you."

Will I ever sing my baby lullabies? Amber anxiously

wondered. Eventually, Amber's voice began to come back. But then, all too soon, it was time for the new mom to return to the hospital for her radiation treatment.

In a Denver hospital, Amber was given the strongest dose of radiation a human can withstand and still live. Then she spent a week in a tiny isolation room without so much as a photograph of Rachel to help wile away the lonely hours. The dose was so strong, no one could come near Amber without exposing themselves to dangerous radiation as well. And trace levels would linger long after Amber got to go home.

"You can't go near your baby until the radiation fades away," the doctor sternly ordered.

Amber felt crushed. "The one thing in the world I want to do most, and you tell me I can't," she anguished.

At home, Amber also had to eat off separate dishes and sit across the living room from the rest of the family on a blanket that would later have to be destroyed. She felt like she'd died and come back as a ghost—always hovering at the very edge of happy family life.

Every day Amber watched from across the room while her mom fed her baby, changed diapers and picked Rachel up when she cried. "Rachel thinks my mom is her mother," she sobbed as she watched her precious little girl happily cooing in Anne's arms. But Amber kept her pain buried deep inside. *My mom has been so wonderful,* she thought. *I couldn't bear it if she felt guilty for helping out.*

But standing at the nursery door listening to her mom sing Rachel to sleep, Amber vividly recalled the day in her car when the baby had started kicking. *It's like my worst nightmare has come true,* she thought. *Someone else is raising my child.*

A few days later, Amber had to fight back tears when Rachel spoke her first word. "Mama," she said, only she said it to her mom instead of to her. *It's been so long. Will my baby ever remember I'm her mother?* Amber wondered.

To Amber, it felt like half a lifetime had gone by, but finally the time arrived when the doctor said she could hold her baby again.

Shortly afterward, Anne returned home. "Thank you, Mom, for everything," Amber said as Jonathan loaded Anne's bags into the car to drive her to the airport.

Amber stayed home with Rachel so she and her baby could become reacquainted. "Come to Mama," she said, but the instant she lifted Rachel into her arms, Amber could tell by the way she fidgeted and turned her head away—her baby had forgotten her. "I finally have my dream to be a mom, only my baby doesn't even know who I am," she sobbed.

Amber was determined to win back her baby. Every day for a month she stretched out on the living-room rug and played peek-a-boo with Rachel. Every night she sang her to sleep in a voice still raspy from her surgery. During the day she hugged her baby and told her again and again how much she loved her. "You mean the world to me," she said, and, slowly, Rachel began to respond.

One day when Rachel lay crying in her playpen, Amber hurried to comfort her. And this time when she picked up her baby she felt the difference. "Mama," Rachel said, and Amber burst into happy tears.

"She knows I'm her mom!" Amber exulted.

Today, five years later, Amber is still cancer free. And Amber is not only Rachel's mom, these days the two are best buddies. They do one another's hair and paint each other's nails. Amber still sings Rachel to sleep with their own, special lullaby every night, and this autumn one of Amber's most cherished dreams came true. "I got to help my little girl get ready for her very first day of kindergarten."

Heather Black

Cute, Cuddly and Calls All the Shots

Nothing I've ever done has given me more joy and reward than being a good father to my children.

Bill Cosby

What would you do if someone told you that a demanding, illogical, selfish, boorish bully was going to move into your home and hold you hostage for the rest of your life?

How would you prepare for the arrival of a person who represents the most basic form of human life—a grunting, drooling, screaming illiterate with absolutely no regard for property or personal hygiene?

Anyone with an ounce of sense would call a cop, maybe the entire SWAT team.

But nobody ever does. Instead, we prepare for these human leeches by knitting booties and sweaters, soliciting gifts and opening bank accounts for them. Some people remodel and furnish rooms for them. Others actually move into bigger homes or apartments.

When it comes to welcoming a new baby, no expense of

time or money is too great to be justified or rationalized, even though that baby is going to make us willing slaves to its everlasting well-being.

If I seem to have a somewhat negative attitude toward parenthood, however, I have given the wrong impression. I love having kids.

But I don't think anyone should enter into such an arrangement without full knowledge of its consequences as well as its benefits.

And according to a survey I read about this week, a lot of people are doing just that. The survey, published in the February edition of *Baby Talk* magazine, says 52 percent of expectant parents don't believe a new baby will change their lifestyle. Another 25 percent say parenting will be easy.

Boy, are they in for a surprise. Because anyone who doesn't think a baby will change his lifestyle is more naive than the infant.

The last time I heard such a statement, it came from a colleague who was about seven months pregnant. "Having a baby won't change our lives *that* much," she insisted. "We won't let it."

Ha-ha! I thought. That is a good one; the assumption that you can "let" or "not let" a baby affect your life. Because once the baby is born, it does the "letting."

The baby lets you sleep or it doesn't, lets you go out for an evening or not. The baby decides whether you can eat your dinner in peace or watch the news or other TV shows, as well as where, when and whether you will take a vacation.

In fact, the baby's needs and your own sense of responsibility to the child will influence nearly every move and decision you make from the day of the baby's birth.

Now that her baby is two years old, my friend is willing to admit how foolish her pre-parental prediction was.

"When I finally sit down at 9:30 or 10:00 at night," she says, "I'm too tired to even think about doing something for myself."

But she still doesn't have all the facts. Because like many others before her—including me—she is operating under the delusion that it will somehow, someday, "get easier."

It doesn't. In fact, it gets harder. So forget about all that freedom you are going to reacquire "when he goes to school," or "when he's old enough to drive himself around" or "when he goes off to college."

Instead, you will do homework, attend PTA meetings and suffer through class plays and other forms of torture. You may become a Scoutmaster, coach, band parent, stage parent or one of many other parental subsets.

What's more, you will pay dearly for all that, not only in time but in currency.

And according to what I've been hearing and reading lately, you don't even get off the hook when they graduate from college or get married. The latest trend—perhaps because of the economy—is for adult children to move back in with their parents.

So the very idea that a child won't change your lifestyle—immediately, drastically and permanently—is a real hoot. Because the fact is that they never leave you alone.

A least, not if you raise them right and have luck on your side.

Ray Recchi

5

SPECIAL DELIVERY

Babies are bits of stardust blown from the hand of God.

   Lucky the women who knows the pangs of birth for she has held a star.

Larry Barretto

A Trusting Love

As I placed the last few items in my suitcase, I could hear the radio playing in our bathroom. My husband, Mark, listened to the news as he shaved every morning. "There are reports of bombing within three miles of the Saigon City limits."

Mark came into the bedroom. We stared into each other's eyes, unable to look away, yet unable to speak. He turned and left the room. When I had agreed to be the next volunteer to escort six babies from Vietnam to their adoptive homes in the United States, there had been no escalation of the war for many months. Still, the decision to leave Mark and our two chubby-cheeked little girls for two weeks was difficult at best. When I asked Mark what he thought I should do, he only said, "You've gotta do what you gotta do, Honey." But I knew the words, "Please, don't go!" were screaming inside him.

I considered how firsthand information would be helpful for our local Friends of Children of Vietnam chapter. Mark and I had applied for adoption of a son through FCVN and expected him in two to three years. I thought it might mean something to our son someday to know his mom had been to his homeland. Every call we made to the State Department gave the same encouraging advice: the war was not expected to escalate. Go. So after much prayer and thought, I said I would. One week later, a fierce Vietcong offensive began. I doubt I'd have kept my promise to go if I hadn't had the powerful, faith-confirming experience on Easter Sunday, the day before I left. I *knew* I'd be safe because God would take care of me.

During the thirty-minute drive to the Cedar Rapids, Iowa, airport, Mark and I hardly spoke. It was strange not to be able to talk about all of this. We had always prided ourselves in our ability to communicate. Mark was not only my husband, but also my confidant, my best friend. There was nothing I couldn't discuss with him—until now.

At the airport, we spent most of my preboarding time wrapped in each other's arms. When the final boarding call was announced, I lingered there a little longer hoping his love and trust for me were greater than his fears.

"I'll assume you're okay unless I hear from the Red Cross," Mark said, knowing phone communication from Vietnam was impossible.

"I'll be fine," I assured him. Still, as I walked across the open concourse to board the plane, I couldn't bring myself to look back and see the pain I knew must be reflected on his face.

Once on board, I forced myself to look out the window and blow him a kiss. He returned it, trying to smile. I leaned back against the seat and allowed the tears to fall.

Days later at my final destination, the Tan San Nhut Airport, the sight of camouflaged jets lining the runway brought to the fore my questions and doubts once again. That is until Cherie, FCVN's Saigon director, greeted me. "Have you heard the news?" she exclaimed. "President Ford has okayed a giant orphan airlift! Instead of taking out six babies, you'll help take out three hundred if we're lucky!"

All the questions were answered; all the doubts, erased.

As she drove through the overcrowded, chaotic streets, Cherie explained how dozens of babies were being brought to the FCVN Center to prepare for the evacuation. Despite my years as a pediatric nurse, I was not ready for what I was about to witness there. Every inch of floor was covered with a mat and every inch of mat was covered with babies! We spent the entire first day helping the Vietnamese workers diaper and feed scores of babbling, cooing, crying infants. Our night's sleep was shattered by the sound of gunfire; harmless, the staff assured us. Still, as glad as I was to be on this mission, I was eager to complete it and get home to Mark and the girls.

So when I learned the next day that FCVN had been bumped from the first place position to leave, I fought to reclaim the right to take the first planeload of orphans to the United States. But to no avail. With disappointment still heavy in our hearts, we instead loaded babies destined for our Australia chapter. With twenty-two babies around me on the floor of a Volkswagen van, we headed to the airport. There we saw an enormous black cloud billowing at the end of the runway. We heard the rumor— the first planeload of orphans, the one I had begged to be on, had crashed after takeoff, killing half of the adults and children onboard.

Stunned, we loaded the babies onto the Australian airliner, then returned to the FCVN Center where the rumor was confirmed. The office was awash with grief. I looked at my watch, still on Iowa time. The girls were having breakfast in their fuzzy pajamas. Mark was shaving and listening to the radio. He would hear the news and be terrified I was on that flight. And there was no way for me to call and spare him this horror and heartache. I slumped onto a rattan sofa and sobbed uncontrollably. Several hours later, the phone rang.

"LeAnn, it's for you," Cherie said. I almost laughed. Who would call me in Saigon? An Associated Press reporter was on the line. A reporter in Iowa had made a series of transpacific calls to reporters covering the war, eventually reaching him, to learn if I had been on the fatal crash. "Sorry to tell you," the journalist said, "the Iowa newsman woke your husband out of a sound sleep to ask him if you were on that plane that crashed. But your husband hadn't heard the morning news yet. We will get this word of your safety to him, I assure you." I began crying again, partly out of sorrow for the grief I was causing Mark, and partly out of joy knowing he'd learn I was all right.

Then, with renewed energy, faith and confidence, I rejoined the workers preparing the babies for our flight— whenever that would be.

The next day at breakfast, Cherie sat beside me. "LeAnn, you and Mark will be adopting one of those babies in the next room. All your paperwork is here and in order. You can wait and be assigned a son from across a desk in the States, or you can go in there now and choose him yourself."

Speechless, I entered the next room and hop-scotched through the sea of babies. Then a little boy, wearing only a diaper, crawled across the floor and into my arms and heart. As I cuddled him, he nestled his head into my shoulder and seemed to hug me back. I carried him around the room, looking at and touching the other babies. I whispered a prayer for the decision I was about to make, knowing it would change many lives forever. "Oh, Mark, I wish you were here." I moaned. "How do I choose?" The little boy in my arms answered by patting my face.

"I know, Son," I whispered. "I love you already, Mitchell."

Two days later, it was our turn to leave. The workers helped us load the babies onto a city bus taking them to their flight to freedom. Nine of us volunteers cared for a hundred babies, placed three and four to a cardboard box. In spite of the stress, it was joyful work as we propped countless bottles and changed diarrhea-soaked diapers. Six hours later, we landed in the Philippines where the

American Red Cross greeted us. "There is no phone access for you here," a grey-haired volunteer said, "But we will call your husband to notify him you're safe." *He'll panic if he gets a call from the Red Cross!* I worried. Patting my hand, the nice lady promised me they would tell him in a manner that would reassure him. I hoped she was right. With a larger plane and more volunteers, we continued the next leg of our journey to Hawaii. There, every child was removed from the plane while it was refueled.

Finally, I could call Mark. The noise around the phone booth was so loud, I had to shout instructions to the operator. I mumbled to myself, "Mark doesn't even know we have a son. He has no idea I'm bringing him home."

I had rehearsed how I would tell him the wonderful news, but when I heard his voice answer the phone, I could only blurt out, "Honey, this is LeAnn," and I started to bawl.

I could hear him repeating my name as he, too, sobbed. I tried to compose myself so I could tell him about Mitchell, but I couldn't catch my breath.

Then, still crying, he said, "Just tell me you're bringing me our son." "Yes! Yes! Yes!" I cried as my heart nearly burst with excitement and love.

When our journey home finally ended, I carried Mitchell across the tarmac of the Cedar Rapids airport. Inside, I was overwhelmed by mobs of reporters with their blinding floodlights and popping flashbulbs. Then Mark stepped through the glare, and Mitchell and I melted into his arms. In Saigon I feared I would never feel his hug again. Now I didn't want to let go. Finally I leaned back so Mark could get a look at his son. Mitchell opened his arms and reached for his daddy. Tears filled Mark's eyes as he hugged him to his chest. Then Mark drew me into the embrace. "Thank you," he whispered.

LeAnn Thieman

Why Our Son Is Named Fox

It was February 1968 and we were expecting our first child. That's a pretty tense moment in any family, but our worries were compounded: My husband Gerry Seldon had just been shipped to Vietnam.

In June of 1967, when we'd first learned of my pregnancy, we were overjoyed. I wanted to have a natural childbirth, so we went faithfully to Lamaze classes, learning to breathe for crunch time, and as my girth increased and my back started aching, Gerry was right there with a pillow just when I needed it. The war was a topic on everyone's mind, but it was happening somewhere else—I was far more interested in what was happening inside me!

And then the unthinkable happened: Gerry got his notice from the draft board; he had to report in a week's time to boot camp. What was I going to do? At first it seemed likely that his draft would be deferred because I was pregnant, but the action was heating up, and as a result of the infamous Tet Offensive, more men were needed on the front

"Don't worry, honey, you know I'm always with you—and I will be back when the baby's due." But I couldn't shake the feeling of disaster. All those hours of coaching and learning how to count and breathe properly! All the times we'd laughed about how Gerry was going to come bravely into the delivery room and then faint at the first sight of blood! How could I go through this without him?

Then I suddenly realized something: I wasn't the only one with an ordeal coming up—and mine was likely to be a good deal safer than his.

Hey, how can I be afraid when I've had such a good coach? Don't worry, I'll be fine!

The next few days passed like a whirlwind. Parties, visiting with his mom and Aunt Louisa and packing. And repacking. I would put some extra pairs of socks in his duffel bag, and he'd surreptitiously sneak them back into his drawer. Then I made some fudge and tried freezing it to put in. That didn't even make it past the bedroom door. Finally he grabbed me into his lap on the bed, laughing. "They're going to give me G.I. clothes anyway, silly!" He promised solemnly that he would write as soon as he got there. On his last day home we went out for dinner, and he gently teased me as we danced one last time: "We don't seem to be as close as we used to, sweetheart."

And then, all of a sudden, he was gone.

His letters from boot camp were full of hilarious stories about his drill sergeant, who seemed to be a walking stereotype, and the mistakes he and some of the other men in his platoon made during drill time. I knew that preparing men for war couldn't be all fun and games, but Gerry never let anything sad filter in.

When boot camp was over, I flew to meet him for a weekend in San Francisco—then, again, he was gone.

Now his letters were much less frequent, but their tone remained the same. It wasn't until much later that I learned that the original ten men of his "Fox" Patrol had become eight, and Gerry himself had come close to being one of the casualties. Names like Saigon, Da Nang, Long

Binh—I hadn't paid much attention to them on the news. But Gerry had been in Long Binh when Bear Cat encampment, a mile down the road, had been overrun and destroyed by the Vietcong.

I tried to do the same: All my letters to him were filled with descriptions of the new mobile Aunt Louisa had given us to hang over the baby's crib, and the little nightshirts and gowns that my sister gave me at my baby shower. Or the time when a mother apologized awkwardly to me in the checkout lane at the supermarket after her six-year-old had gazed curiously at me and asked (in a very loud voice), "How come that lady's so fat, Mommy?" I told Gerry how ponderous I was getting, but I never mentioned how I'd wake up at night when the baby kicked me and roll over to show him—only to feel the cold bed and the empty pillow.

There were precious moments when Gerry's platoon was in a secure place, and the men were allowed to call home. The nine minutes that each man was allotted always seemed to fly by in as many seconds, but his voice always drew us together and made it seem as if he were actually by my side.

With Gerry gone, my father- and mother-in-law tried extra hard to make me feel secure and safe, but it wasn't the same, of course. When my labor started in the middle of an icy February night, I called them.

"Sorry to wake you, Dad—I think it's time you came over. I'm fine, but I'm pretty sure I should go to the hospital." He was there so fast that I suspect he'd taken to going to bed with his clothes on and his car keys in his hand—and for once in his life, my father-in-law exceeded the speed limit. When he handed me over to the care of the nurse at the admitting desk, I could almost hear his sigh of relief.

From that moment on, things were a blur. Hours went by, and figures in brightly colored clothes kept saying cheerily, "You're doing fine." Right. All I could think of was "I want my husband." The doctor was saying, "Now breathe, you remember, just like you did in class." I tried, but without Gerry to coach me and hold my hand, I couldn't seem to get the hang of it. The baby seemed to be feeling his absence, too, because with all our efforts, he seemed very reluctant to be born.

And then the miracle occurred. A nurse came up to the table with a phone, and held it up to my ear. It was Gerry! Knowing this was my due date, he'd called home, and my mother-in-law had given him the hospital number. Even while my head whirled with the excitement of hearing his voice, a small mental voice was saying "You only have nine minutes—only nine minutes. He's going to hang up soon, and you'll be alone again."

But I made the most of those nine minutes. "Breathe," said Gerry, and I would breathe and push as he counted. "Breathe." Dr. O'Connell seemed very pleased.

Maybe I *was* doing fine! All at once I had the strange sensation that Gerry's voice had been multiplied and somewhat amplified. And certainly more than nine minutes had passed? I stole a look at the hands of the large clock that hung on the wall. It had been over an hour since Gerry first called. *I must be hallucinating!* I glanced at the nurse's face, and she was smiling—but crying, too. What was happening? When I realized the truth, I burst out laughing.

Each of the men of Fox Patrol had surrendered his nine minutes so that Gerry could be with me when our son was born, but only with the understanding that they could take part. Instead of having one husband coaching me through my labor, I had eight G.I.'s yelling "Breathe! 1-2-3-4 . . ." into the phone!

"Okay, one more big push." I was awfully tired, but as I gathered myself for another effort, Dr. O'Connell's command was echoed by all the men of Fox Patrol, and when my son made his entrance into the world, the warm congratulations of the delivery room staff were drowned by cheers and yells from the other side of the world!

Our initial impulse was to name him Gerald Luis Tyrone William Javier Chico Sung Li Carl Seldon, after all the men who had helped bring our son into the world. Then our common sense took over, and we took pity on the boy who would have to write his full name so many times in his life.

And *that's* why our son is named Fox.

Mary Jane Strong

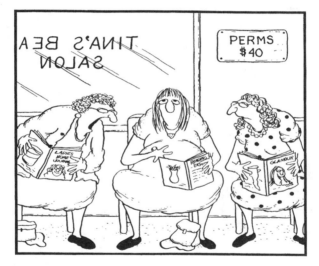

"That's nothing, I've got a friend who was in labor for sixty-seven hours, she couldn't take any medication because she's allergic, and in the midst of it all the entire maternity staff went on strike and her baby had to be delivered by a janitor."

Baby on Board

All of us are born for a reason, but all of us don't discover why. Success in life has nothing to do with what you gain in life or accomplish for yourself. It's what you do for others.

Danny Thomas

Sandy and Theresa de Bara of Greenfield Park, New York, decided to take their three-year-old daughter, Amanda, to Disney World. They wanted to give her a special treat before the arrival of their new baby, who wasn't due for two months.

The morning they were to leave for Orlando, Theresa called her doctor complaining of "indigestion and a little pressure." But he told her that it was probably false labor, which she had experienced with Amanda.

Shortly after the plane took off, Theresa doubled over in pain. She knew this was no indigestion. This was labor. Sandy flagged down flight attendant Meg Somerville, and once Somerville realized what was happening, she cleared a five-seat row so Theresa could lie down.

Then Somerville got on the public-address system and

said, "We have a woman in labor. If there is a physician on board, please report to row twenty-eight."

Steven Rachlin, M.D., an internist from Old Brookville, New York, who was also taking his family to Disney World, sprang to Theresa's side. He had delivered a baby just once before—which had been thirteen years earlier.

After a quick examination, he saw that Theresa was bleeding. "I see the head starting to crown," he announced to Somerville. "This lady is having the baby right now!"

While flight attendants scurried to get blankets, the pilot radioed controllers at Dulles International Airport near Washington, D.C., to tell them he needed to make an emergency landing. Sandy stood helplessly off to the side, praying that his wife and the baby would pull through. A woman traveling with her own children soon took charge of Amanda, who was sobbing and asking if her mother was going to die.

As the plane began its emergency descent, Theresa gave birth. But the baby, a boy, arrived with his umbilical cord wrapped around his neck. He had turned blue and wasn't breathing.

Rachlin started CPR, massaging the newborn's chest with two fingers and shouting, "Breathe, baby, breathe!"

"God," moaned Theresa, "please save his life!"

Just then, two other passengers, James and Jen Midgley of Chelmsford, Massachusetts, who were both paramedics as well as being husband and wife, offered to help the failing baby. Jen's specialty is infant respiratory procedure. She turned to the flight attendants and said, "We need a straw!"

"We don't carry any on board," replied one of the crew members. But attendant Denise Booth had brought a juice box with her; it had a straw attached to the side.

While Rachlin continued CPR, Jen carefully steered the straw down the infant's throat. Then she suctioned fluid out of the infant's lungs. Finally, after five nerve-jangling minutes, the baby began to cry. A shoelace donated by a passenger was used to tie off the umbilical cord. As the baby's wailing filled the cabin, everyone on board clapped and cheered.

Once the plane had landed, waiting paramedics whisked mother and baby to nearby Reston Hospital Center. As Theresa was carried away, the passengers gave her a standing ovation. Sandy hugged Steven Rachlin, and everyone cheered again.

After an hour on the ground, the plane took off for Orlando with free drinks for all the passengers. Before they arrived, the captain announced that the baby—named Matthew Dulles, after the emergency landing site—was holding his own at the hospital's special-care nursery. Theresa was also doing fine.

As it turned out, though, Matthew had respiratory problems. He remained in the hospital for three weeks before being allowed to go home.

"There are just no words to thank everyone," Sandy told reporters later. "People in Virginia invited us into their homes, baby-sat Amanda, even offered to do our laundry. And an Alaskan hockey team sent Matthew equipment. They said anyone who could survive that birth is strong enough to play their game."

Amanda was too young to understand much about what had happened. All she knew was that during the flight, Mommy had a bellyache, Matthew was born and a lot of people were running around.

But the little girl did take away one interesting insight from the whole episode. "Now I know where babies come from," she said afterward.

"Where?" she was asked.

"Airplanes!"

Allan Zullo and John McGran

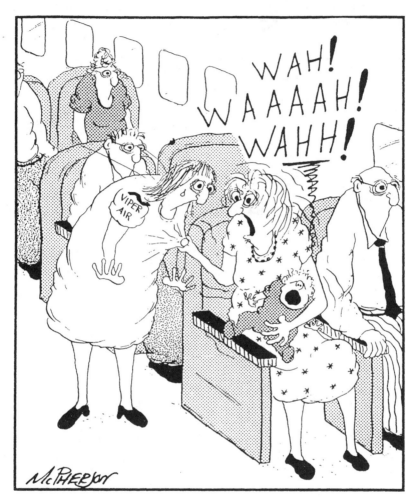

"I don't think you understand! I said, 'The pacifier fell out somewhere back in the airport!' Tell the pilot to turn the plane around—now."

Baby Mall

My husband brought our three young children down the long hall of the maternity ward, pausing to let them wave in each doorway at the new mothers cuddling bundles. At my room, he beckoned them in and introduced them to their new brother.

Five-year-old Katrina gingerly fingered the baby's thick red hair that the nurse had brushed and oiled into a fat top curl. She inspected his little feet, admired his tiny ears, and planted kisses on his dimpled elbow. But her coos stopped short at his wrist.

Drawing back, she pointed at the identification bracelet and frowned, "Look, Mommy. They left the price tag on!"

Carol McAdoo Rehme

Pre-Parenthood

The social worker is due in a few hours. We're basically ready. I mean, we've cleaned this house like nobody's business. And we've put rock salt all over the driveway so she won't slip. I was going to make applesauce so the house would have the warm, welcoming smell of cinnamon. But now I'm thinking I should bake bread instead. Or how about a fire in the fireplace? The smell of a fire definitely says: Home.

But what is the smell of Parent? More specifically, what is the smell of Good Parent Material? The social worker is coming to consider us. She's coming to our house today to do a "home study," step one in the adoption procedure.

Alex and I have decided to adopt a baby from China. Well, we haven't *decided* decided, but we're deep into the decision process. The deeper you go, the more your heart starts pounding.

There's a lot you can do before you commit. Lots of paperwork you can get behind you. So this is what we are doing. This is our way of deciding, of tiptoeing, of cracking open the door to the unknown.

"Do you think we should have the smell of baking bread wafting through the house?" I ask Alex.

"Might be a little contrived," he says. "We never bake bread."

"Okay applesauce."

"We don't make that either," he says.

"I made it in seventh grade," I point out. "It was the first thing we cooked in home ec."

"All right," he says. He knows to surrender when I am being driven by stress.

"But will the smell get all the way back to the family room?" I ask. "Should we bring a fan in here or something and aim the aroma toward the back of the house?"

"No," he says. "No—we should not." He knows to speak clearly, definitively, when I am losing my marbles.

I'm nervous. I've never had a home study before. I've never had to put my domestic self out for review. It is not my most developed self. My inner Martha Stewart is not what you'd call a fully actualized identity.

It doesn't help that it's raining. That the ice outside is slowly giving way to a yard that looks like soup. "Welcome to the ugliest day on our farm!" I imagine saying to her when she pulls up. But then she might think I mean it's ugly because she's here, so no, I'd better not go there.

I'm nervous. I want this to go right. I'm peeling apples. I'm wiping the counters again and again to show off what a good counter wiper I am. I am sprinkling cinnamon on the apples, lots of it to make sure the aroma of my own domesticity, of my promise as a mother, is unmistakable.

I could, of course, be insulted. I mean, maybe that's the more empowering emotional direction to go in right now. The outrage! A home study? Why should I have to prove my parental potential to a complete stranger? Any wacko with the right plumbing can make himself or herself a parent. No forms to fill out. No history to reveal. No how-do-you-handle-conflict essay questions to answer. Why me? Poor me. It's not fair. Life isn't fair. Which, of course is only half the story. Life seems unfair only when it's throwing curves. But what about when it's sending out those equally rare perfect pitches, a good job, a good husband, a happy home, a supportive family, a baby who needs a mom. In China, we're told that would be a girl.

Okay, here comes a car. A white car. Make that a muddy white car. Oh, dear I should have prepared her. She pulls up the driveway, sits there for a few minutes. She's flipping through papers, writing things down. She's giving us bad marks for mud. I can just tell. I am biting my nails. I am pacing.

"Just be yourself," Alex says. He has an umbrella. He is going outside to her.

"Brilliant move!" I say. "Bring her an umbrella! Blind her with chivalry!"

"It's raining," he says.

When she gets in the house I begin my apologies. For the rain. For the gray sky. For the ruts on Wilson Road. For the way the kitchen is not yet renovated. For the light bulb that is out on the porch. For the way the cat sleeps in the satellite dish receiver despite the fact that I have provided him with a perfectly good cat bed.

"You seem nervous," she says, smiling. "Please don't be. This is not an investigation. This is a . . . warm-and-fuzzy. You know? I'm just here to help you bring your daughter home."

My . . . what? Excuse me? This is the first time I have ever heard that word used that way. That is one big word. "Daughter." "My daughter." "Our daughter." That has a ring to it all right. Alex looks at me. He is smiling. I am smiling. The social worker is smiling. Three people enjoying the same music. Decisions are like music. New songs you try out. The more beautiful the sound, the more your hearts starts pounding.

Jeanne Marie Laskas

The Labors of Love

Childbirth is difficult, but holding the child makes the pain worthwhile.

Marianne Willamson

I'm not sure, but I'm almost certain, that I'm the first woman to give birth. At least that's how I felt last September, when Catlyne was born.

Even the word "daughter" fills me with the most enormous sense of pride. And though there are hundreds of thousands of daughters out there, I can't help feeling that I had the first "real" one. The truth of the matter is that an emotional door was opened that I never knew existed. However, you couldn't have convinced me of this during labor.

How come all the women in my life who had so graciously shared countless stories about titanic weight gain, heartburn, swollen feet, nausea and other charming side effects of pregnancy never got around to telling me about labor? If someone told me how much it was going to hurt, I could've backed out of the whole deal while there was still time.

The Lamaze class we snickered through suddenly became a priceless source of information when labor began. . . . I knew what kind of anesthetics to ask for (or demand in this case), which I did ask (demand) for the minute I arrived on the labor floor. The problem is, however, anesthetics aren't given until you've dilated to five centimeters (for all of you who haven't experienced this "miracle of life" you don't get the prize until you've hit ten). I was certain that with all the pain I was going through, I must have reached at least eight. I was informed by a nurse with a funny smile that I was at one.

I wanted to hit her. Hard.

So I waited nearly ten hours, and during that time I started to think. They say there's a reason for everything, even the most painful things in life. I know this is true, and during the pain I had a divine revelation: God is not a woman.

No woman would put another human being through that kind of torture. She would have designed a woman's body in a more thoughtful way. At least she would have devised an equally agonizing experience for men to live through—to sort of even things out.

You know, the nine months of pregnancy weren't too bad. I made it through three months of feeling like throwing up, a disappearing waist and completely eliminating sleeping on my back if I wanted to breathe at the same time. I didn't mind foregoing beer (well, maybe a little), or anything else that's bad for you but tastes good. I packed away my cute bikini undies in exchange for underwear that went to my chin and bought a "nice" cotton bra forty-seven sizes bigger than my nice lace ones. All this I figured was worth it.

But not labor. That is, until I saw her head.

No one could have prepared me for the overwhelming rush of emotion I felt when I saw this tiny human being. I

never loved anyone as much as I loved her. Any incon-
venience or discomfort seemed so small and insignificant
compared to the miracle I was looking at.

It's funny. No one in the world could have convinced
me that I would feel this wonderful about having a baby.
I'm from the thirty-something generation of women
determined to have careers and lives different from our
mothers. No way was I going to stay home and take care
of four children and one man the rest of my life. I refused
to learn anything which I felt was remotely domestic.
Marriage and children evoked nothing but feelings of
entrapment. I liked being single, working, traveling and
taking care of myself.

When I thought of having children, I was prepared for
bottles, dirty diapers, crying and a lifetime of responsibility.
But I forgot about the human being part. It never occurred
to me that a child could bring love to your life and the
responsibility to care for her would be a pleasure. It's nice
to care for someone else besides myself for a change.

Catlyne has affected all of us. Father is happier. He's
taking better care of himself so he will be around to teach
her how to play softball. My sister has practically moved
in with us in hope that if she stays long enough, she'll get
custody of the baby on the basis of homestead rights. We
all smile more, laugh more, love each other more. How
come nobody told me how great this would be?

So what's a little pain?

Claire Simon Laisser

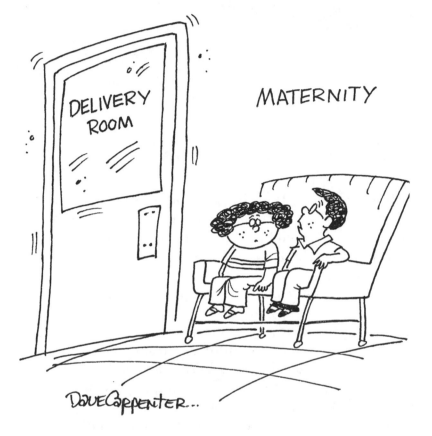

"Boy that stork sure can scream."

Two for One

Early in the autumn of 1983, as the leaves began to change, the air became crisp and my belly began to "show" my fifth child growing inside me, my hopes for birthing this child were dashed during a routine O.B. checkup.

No heartbeat could be detected, and an ultrasound showed I had a blighted ovum. My doctor scheduled a D & C for the following week.

I chose my words carefully, as I tried to explain to my oldest child, seven-year-old Elisa, that this belly of mine, just beginning to show, wasn't going to grow into a baby as her brothers and sister had.

I felt so inadequate, so empty that winter, but the energies emanating from four young children, plus the bonus of some heavy snowfalls kept me busy making snow forts and of course, "angels in the snow." Still, I longed to become pregnant again as soon as possible.

Just after the New Year, my doctor confirmed what I had suspected for several weeks: Yes, I was indeed expecting again. I was sent home with a due date of mid-September and ordered to take it easy.

Arriving home from my doctor's appointment, and

anxious to tell the kids the good news, all I could get out of my mouth was "Guess what, guys?"

Before I could say anything else, Elisa interrupted with, "You're gonna have a baby!" She continued with wide-eyed excitement, "But, you're gonna have two babies, because God took that last one away to heaven!"

"Whoa," I said, "Hold on! It doesn't work that way. Twins don't run in our family."

"But, Mom!" she persisted, "I just know that you're gonna have two babies, and they will be girls with blonde hair and they will look just alike!"

Well, there was no persuading her otherwise, plus she had pretty well convinced her brothers and sister.

I thought what she had said was pretty cute, so I laughed and joked about it to family and friends, and my belly grew and grew.

Soon, these friends that had laughed with me were saying, "Ya know, maybe she is right; you're really getting big!" But I would always say, "No, no, the doctor says there is only one in there."

Because of my now "really big belly" my doctor scheduled an ultrasound, thinking maybe I had miscalculated, and perhaps my due date was sooner than originally thought.

July 6, 1984, as I lay on a gurney ready to explode because I had to drink five glasses of water, the technician began to scan my mountainous belly.

"Well, here's a head, an arm, a leg, and this baby has a good strong heartbeat," she told me, but she was only on the right side of my stomach. Naïve little me asked, "But what is this over here?" She matter-of-factly said, "We'll look at that one next." She must have noticed the shocked look on my face, because she said, "You didn't know you were carrying twins?"

I about fell off the table! As she continued to scan, pointing out various body parts, and finally saying they were both probably girls and most likely identical, I kept hearing Elisa in my head saying, "See, I told you so!"

Needless to say, when I broke the "news" to my husband that evening, he wore a pathway on the carpet (just as I thought he would). And just as I knew she would, Elisa was jumping up and down saying, "See, I told you so! I just knew it!"

We spent the next several weeks watching. My belly grew out of control, and the babies exercising and wiggling around, finding a comfortable position in my crowded womb, became the main source of entertainment each evening.

At last, on August 24, 1984, a couple of weeks before their expected due date, identical twin girls, Sarah and Julie arrived.

The first time Elisa saw them, in her quiet voice as she gently stroked their faces and held their little hands, she said, "See Mom, I told you so! God took that other baby to heaven, and I just knew he was gonna give us two baby girls that look just alike and here they are!"

It's been fifteen years since their birth, and I still tell this story about how the twins came to be. And yes, I guess twins really do run in the family, because Elisa is now also the mother of two-year-old twins! See, Elisa, I told you so!

Elisabeth Sartorius

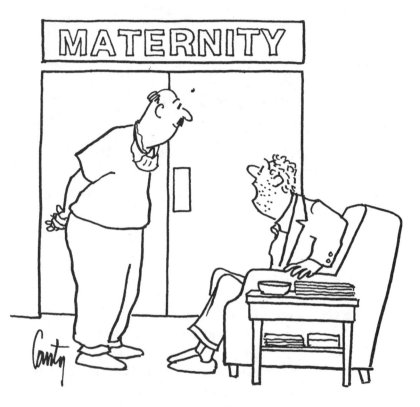

"No, she wasn't on fertility drugs. Why?"

Our Story

No one has ever measured, not even poets, how much the heart can hold.

Zelda Fitzgerald

When we first walked into the restaurant, my husband, Mike, asked me which one "she" was? In my always loving, supportive voice, I said, "I imagine that she is the pregnant girl sitting over there." We were walking into what could be the most important day of our marriage to that point. We were going to meet a prospective birth mother.

Mike and I had been married and "trying" for several years. Friends and acquaintances had given us their pregnancy advice. We had tried and failed with several fertility doctors. We were told to relax, to move this way and that way and—my all-time favorite—to lie in pine! I imagined us relaxed, pine needles thrown everywhere, and a rash, not fertility close at hand. Needless to say, none of these ideas led to pregnancy.

One night, we sat down and discussed what was important to us. Together, we knew that we wanted to be a mom and a dad to someone who we could love unconditionally.

It didn't matter how the child came into the world but what we did after the child was here. Adoption seemed like the perfect option for us, and we thought deciding would be all it took. Boy, were we wrong!

We began our adoption journey with an adoption counselor. The adoption counselor asked us to make a photocopied booklet of our family together and to write a cover letter about our desire to adopt. The letter was to begin, "Dear Birth Mother."

It was difficult to find the perfect way to word letter. We knew that it took amazing strength and love for any woman to consider adoption. A woman who was considering adoption wanted what was best for her child, not necessarily what was best for herself. We found it impossible to put our overwhelming feelings and desires into a one-page letter. It took us weeks to compile our thoughts and write a letter that we were never fully satisfied with.

After we had completed our initial paperwork, our adoption counselor matched us with a girl who was several months pregnant. She already had a daughter and was living at home with her mother. She said that adoption would be the best for everyone. I was hooked, but Mike was leery. We spent hours talking on the telephone and corresponding by letter. We were the couple for her!

Her daughter was born on April eleventh and on April twelfth, she changed her mind. We were devastated, but we understood.

One Saturday, I went to an infertility meeting. A woman from an adoption agency was there and discussed her nonprofit, Christian-based organization. This representative said that the agency stayed with adoptive couples until a child was placed in the home. When I returned home, Mike and I talked about the agency and decided to give adoption another try.

The new agency had us complete a home study

involving bundles of paperwork and several home visits. It was not the nightmarish invasion of privacy that we had heard about. We prepared a booklet and a cover letter with this agency too. Our new adoption journey began and led us with a telephone call to the restaurant.

Walking over to the table, I felt my knees buckle. Minutes ago, I had been ravenous, but now I no longer wanted to eat. Mike and I sat across from a young, pretty pregnant girl and her social worker. We exchanged first names, made small talk and ordered lunch.

The young girl asked us about becoming parents. I remember that I was so filled with emotion that at the word parent I began to cry. She stood up, said she would be back in a minute and left. My husband glanced my way as if to say, "Did you have to cry?"

In a few minutes that passed by like hours, she returned. She was holding two sonogram pictures. She told us that she wanted us to be her daughter's parents. I don't know how someone feels when they win the lottery and think that their dreams may come true, but I can guess.

On the drive home, I asked Mike what he thought. He told me that it sounded wonderful, but we would have to wait and see. The baby was due in a month. The month passed slowly. We waited by the telephone to hear from the adoption agency. When the agency called, they told us that the baby had turned and that a C-section would be performed on Friday. It was Monday. We would be parents within days!

On Friday, my mother drove with us to the hospital. My stepfather stayed at home with our dog. I remember being in a state of airy disbelief. Reality wasn't within my realm.

Walking into the hospital room, we saw the baby lying peacefully on the birth mother's stomach. She immediately asked us if we wanted to hold her.

The baby was the most beautiful creature I had ever laid eyes on. Her head was perfectly round, her body petite and she didn't cry when I cradled her in my arms. Holding her, I thought the birth mother would certainly change her mind. As if knowing what I was thinking, the birth mother said, "If you're thinking what I think you're thinking, please don't. I won't change my mind."

The baby was to be released on Sunday. The birth mother wanted to spend time with her daughter. Everyone thought this wasn't a good idea because she would certainly change her mind. I thought it was such a small request for what she was allowing us to do for the rest of our lives.

The birth mother cried, held and loved the baby that weekend. At one point, she called the head nurse in to talk. We were told this was a sure sign that she wanted to raise the baby herself. The birth mother and the head nurse spoke for what seemed like hours.

The birth mother never wavered in her decision. On Sunday afternoon, my mom, Mike and I walked slowly out of the hospital and a nurse handed us our daughter. What an incredibly joyous moment!

Mike and I have been parents for over six years now. We never knew how much our hearts would be filled with love for a child. Being parents is a most fulfilling way to live. We never forget the love that sent us on our parental journey—the love of a birth mother for her daughter that allowed us to become parents. We thank her in prayer and a story that we share with our daughter about her birth. Birth mothers are truly the most courageous, loving individuals that we know. There's one in particular that we hold in highest esteem.

Judy Ryan

Letting Go

Only mothers can think of the future, because they give birth to it in their children.

Maxim Gorky

When I found out I was going to have twins, my husband and I were thrilled. We felt that God had answered our prayers. So when I started to go into labor at only twenty-four weeks along, I was devastated. I threw myself into cocooning around the two too-small children. I obeyed every doctor's order. I stayed in bed twenty-four hours a day. When I was hospitalized, I prayed every day. I tried to meditate myself into a state of peacefulness that the babies would respond to, and perhaps slow down their rush into the world. I was determined to prevent these children from making the mistake of coming into the world too soon.

So when it became clear that labor was inevitable, that nothing I could do would prevent the babies from coming, I was thrown into a panic. My body shook with the pain of guilt and regret. I blamed myself. How could I care for them as children when my body had failed to care for them as fetuses? How could I create an environment for them where they wouldn't be hurt, where they would be safe always?

I dozed on and off throughout the early part of labor. I dreamed of a visitor who came in and out of my room. The visitor held my hand, stroked my forehead and spoke to me. I felt tears stinging my eyes as the visitor spoke, but I immediately recognized the truth of what was said. I woke to find myself alone in the room, the monitors pinging away as they counted the twin beats of my babies' hearts.

I grabbed my journal and quickly began to write a letter to my soon-to-be-born sons. Right then and there, I gave them their freedom to do whatever they needed to do. I told them that I loved them, that I hoped they would want to stay near us, and that I would do whatever I could to help them through their lives. Tears flowed freely as I read the letter out loud to them. I told them, in a rush of words, that life was in their hands now, not mine. I released them from my needs, my hopes and my dreams for them. They could choose what to do. I was heartbroken and exhilarated as I spoke, anxious to see them, terrified to lose them. But it was their choice.

A strange peace settled over me as I finished speaking. My hands fluttered softly over my swollen belly as I said good-bye to the little ones that I had carried for seven months. "It's okay, whatever you choose is okay. I love you. I love you."

Moments later, an intense contraction hit, sweeping over me in a wave of pure energy. The force of the labor pains crescendoed, and I knew there was no turning back. I felt the silent visitor near me again, holding me, helping me as nurses came and went. My husband arrived, and stayed near me, silent and grim. "Honey," I said, "It's okay, it's up to them now." He nodded, not really understanding, and gripped my hand tighter.

The boys were whisked quickly into intensive care upon their arrival into the world. They stayed there, fighting for life, for two months. I helped them, I cheered them on, I loved them. I sat for hours, telling them what life might be like with us, here on earth. I hoped they listened. I prayed they listened. But it was clear, even then, that they were their own men. All I could do was wait and watch the drama of their lives unfold.

As I write this, I am again faced with the pain of letting them go. Of course, the exhilaration is there, too. I am glad for my silent guide's comforting presence as I watch my now six-foot sons stand to accept their high school diplomas. Tears flow freely as I wonder if they are ready, if I have done enough to prepare them for their lives. Michael is preparing to do community service work in Fiji. Will he be all right? Jack is going on to study music; he has been playing classical guitar since he was five. Will he ever find a job? My husband squeezes my hand. He's read my mind. He leans in and whispers to me, "Honey, it's okay, it's up to them now." I nod, not really understanding, and grip his hand tighter.

They march past me, laughing and whispering to each other in the way that only twins can. Finally, I catch their attention. "Hi, Mom," Michael says, raising his diploma in celebration. "Did you ever think we'd make it?" Jack laughs and grabs his shoulder as they go out to join their classmates.

"Yes," I think. "Oh, yes. I always knew you'd make it."

Kate Andrus

$\overline{6}$

SMALL MIRACLES

Love the moment, and the energy of that moment will spread beyond all boundaries

Sister Corita Kent

Blessed Laughter

Sarah said, "God has brought me laughter, and everyone who hears about this will laugh with me."

Genesis 21:6

It had been an unusually quiet evening in our obstetrics unit. After weeks of numerous deliveries and nonstop busyness, the last of our postpartum patients and their newborns had been discharged. With no patients, our nurse aides had floated to other areas where they were needed, and me and Karen, the other scheduled nurse, were all that remained in our department.

We were enjoying the quiet for a change when the phone rang.

"That was Cindy in ER," Karen said, as she hung up the phone. "She says they're sending someone back who *may* be in labor." She paused, grinning slightly.

"What?" I pressed.

"Well, Cindy said the woman and her husband didn't even know they were pregnant!"

I raised my eyebrows quizzically, but before I found words to respond, the maternity room doors burst open.

An emergency room stretcher, carrying a heavy-set woman in her mid-forties, pushed by a harried ER nurse, barreled down the hallway toward us. An older man was trotting alongside, holding her hand. Both were red-faced and panting heavily, she to delay giving birth, he in an attempt to keep up.

We sprang into action and quickly moved her to a labor bed while the ER nurse beat a hasty retreat. A quick check of the woman proved that she was indeed very pregnant and very much in labor. She had labored to the point of being fully dilated and was already feeling the strong urge to push. Not having known she was pregnant, she had no obstetrician. So, while I finished prepping her and instructing her on breathing techniques, Karen called emergency to borrow one of their resident doctors to deliver her. Otherwise, we would soon be performing the honor ourselves!

Less than half an hour later, the woman gave birth to a vigorous, yowling, though very small, baby girl.

After the infant had been pronounced healthy by the resident doctor, I cleaned and diapered her. Then the swaddled baby was returned to her parents, and Karen and I finally had time to find out how the mother could have missed that she was pregnant. This was Ellen and Jake's story:

She and Jake had gone bowling that evening. While she was taking her turn with the ball, she suddenly experienced what she described as "intense abdominal cramping." She tried to ignore it at first, but it increased in intensity, persisting to the point that she was convinced she was having a gallbladder attack.

Similar symptoms had appeared to a lesser degree over the past several months. At first, her doctor felt it was heartburn. Later, he considered other digestive problems; she was prescribed antacids and urged to watch her stress levels and cut down on fatty foods. Finally, her doctor attributed the recurring problem to gallstones.

"But why wasn't pregnancy ever considered?" Karen asked boldly.

Ellen laughed through her tears, tenderly stroking the cherub cheek of her brand new daughter. "We've tried for over fifteen years. Every test there is, I've had. So has Jake. We were simply told it was impossible, that we couldn't have babies."

Her balding husband, still in shock and speechless, just shook his head and grinned as he caressed the soft strawberry blonde hair on his daughter's tiny head with his big leathery knuckle.

"And then," she went on, "when my monthlies stopped, I figured, well, The Change, you know. After all, I am old enough for that. My doctor thought so, too. And Jake and I finally accepted that it just wasn't meant to be."

Ellen's eyes brightened as she gently rocked her baby, then bent to kiss her daughter's sweet-smelling head. "Oh Lord, thank you, thank you! How we've so wanted a baby all these years, and now you've blessed us with one!" She looked up at her husband. "Jake, we have a baby! And look how beautiful she is!"

The rest of that shift, Karen and I laughed and cried with the new parents, sharing in their unexpected joy. This was over twenty years ago, yet I can still hear Jake and Ellen's joyful laughter. I can still hear their heartfelt thanks to the Lord for his most blessed gift of love to them.

Like an earthly father, with a twinkle in his eye, who delighted in surprising his children with a very special gift, so God had surprised this humble couple with this most extraordinary one.

And, since that evening, besides believing more than ever that God still performs miracles, I also wholeheartedly believe this: God most definitely has a sense of humor. After all, Ellen and Jake just thought they were going out for a night of bowling!

Susanna Burkett Chenoweth

Grandpa's Precious Gift

I wanted a baby with all my heart, but I was not getting pregnant. I waited, I prayed, I cried and I went to my parents when I could not find any more courage inside myself. With their love and support, I carried on . . . through tests, artificial insemination, in vitro fertilization and life in general.

Over four years passed. Then, on March 8, 1997, a day I will never forget, my loving father passed away. He was our leader. He believed in us more than we did. He believed in miracles. Our family felt lost without him. My mom, my siblings and I all struggled, trying to keep our spirits up without Dad by our side. All the while, I kept trying for a baby, to no avail. I finally surrendered all my trust over to God's hands in order to find some peace in my heart. On a television show, my mom saw a speaker who suggested writing a letter to your deceased love one to help heal your wounds. Unbeknownst to me, she tried it and it seemed to help her immensely.

After five long years of trying to conceive, it finally happened. I was pregnant! My baby's due date was the day before my dad's birthday. Yet, that day came and went. My baby girl, Samantha, decided to be born right on her grandpa's sixty-first birthday! What an extra wonderful surprise. When it seemed like one door closed in my life, somehow it was opened right back up.

When Samantha was about six months old, I continued to marvel at the miracle of hope I had been given from heaven. It was then that my mom told me about her letter to dad. Here is the part she wrote about me. "Sharon and Ron still have had no luck on having a little one. Maybe you can ask God to give them some help!" That letter was written two months before I got pregnant.

I am writing this letter to my mom, dad and, of course, God as thanks for keeping my heart full of love, hope, trust and the strength to believe in miracles. Also, thanks from Samantha—Grandpa's precious gift.

Sharon Crismon

My Father's Tears

My dad was always the strong silent type. Growing up, I rarely saw him angry, or even raise his voice in debate. He was often miserable with allergies, but didn't take it out on us. He never told me he loved me, that just was not his way. This was difficult for me growing up.

I remember one time I cried and cried. Finally my mother reached out and comforted me. Then my father said "the words." When you have to put up a fuss to hear someone say "I love you," it makes the words feel empty and of little consolation.

Yet deeply buried and hidden inside me was the knowledge that he loved me. Even though he was hard to get to know, I remember finding the key to opening him up a little. Only when working next to him, would he talk more freely. Through all these growing up years, I never saw him cry.

Years later, my first son, his first grandson was born. He was born in the dark, cold, early morning hours of a winter blizzard.

Still exhausted and scared, I called my parents. With the storm still raging, they could only "try to make it" the next day.

My husband and I were both students and very poor. We had no means to pay the hospital, so I had a very limited stay. Exhausted and numb from the emotional waves of ecstasy and despair, I longed to stay longer.

Late in the afternoon of the next day, my roommate left for a walk and snack. I had the sleeping baby with me. I tried to sleep, but could not. I startled at the sound of light knocking. The nurse peeked in.

"I know it isn't visiting hours," she said, "but, this is a special visitor," then she disappeared.

There was my dad, standing in the doorway and looking terribly out of place. He had a blue carnation in a small white vase tied with a blue ribbon. I guessed he picked it up at the hospital gift shop. He was still in his dirty old work coat. The dirt on his hands and face told me he came straight from work.

He looked at me sheepishly as he crept a little way into the room. My eyes meet his.

I saw a tear in is eye. It welled up, and gently rolled down his cheek. And then another. And another.

I never saw my father cry before—the silent emotion was overwhelming. "See your grandson?" I blurted out trying to hide my own feeling of awkwardness. But it was useless. Tears glazed over my eyes as well.

Then we were both in tears, as he gingerly made his way closer and handed me the carnation. He slowly stretched to peek at the baby—keeping his distance. He stayed only briefly. Then he was gone.

Although few words were spoken that visit, it touched me deeply. I knew beyond any doubt that my father loved me, and was proud of me. Those tears will forever be in my heart.

Robin Clifton

Miracle of Life

For the last few years on Mother's Day I find myself thinking of a woman I only knew for a brief time when I was very young, but who would have a lasting impression with me and my family.

The story goes back to when I was eleven years old. We lived in the city of Albany, New York, and at the time, my parents rented the top floor of one of those typical old three-story city houses, joined by mutual walls on both sides and forming rows of brick buildings, like cutouts or clones, on both sides of long streets. There was a "flat," as the apartments were than called, under us and another in the basement.

The owners lived in the basement. They were a lovely older Italian couple with a few grown children. One of their sons had recently married and he and his wife lived in the middle flat.

My job that summer was to take care of my little brother Joey, then three years old. I could take him to the nearby park during the day, but could never stay away too long. My mother would get nervous if she didn't see us after a couple of hours. So I would bring Joey home and let him play on his tricycle up and down the sidewalk parallel to the house where we lived.

Many a time I was fiercely bored, but in those days of authoritarian parents and obedient kids, I knew better than to complain. One thing that helped a lot was being able to spend some time with my neighbor on the second floor, now a young and happy mother-to-be.

They called her "Catuzza" which meant, my father told me, sweet little Catherine. The ". . . uzza" was a diminutive that Italians put at the end of a name when a child was particularly sweet and it usually stuck into adulthood. And she was, indeed, sweet. She was also beautiful and I loved to be near her.

Catuzza was well into her pregnancy that summer, and it was evident that she was often lonely. She knew very little English and during the day missed her husband a great deal. He was a shoemaker and worked long hours to provide for his budding family. She enjoyed the company of myself and Joey. My little brother had golden curls which she would twine around her fingers. Her smile would always make me feel that she was wondering about her own child, in her womb.

Sometimes when the baby would kick, she would let me touch her stomach, and once, when Joey was close by, he, too, put his hand on her, much to her embarrassment. In those days, children weren't supposed to know about babies being in a mother's tummy.

As summer came to an end, we made plans to move to another flat in another area of the city. My mother, who always got bored with where we lived, simply decided to move as she had almost every year that I could remember. I never saw Catuzza again until just a few years ago.

My brother Joe grew up to join the U.S. Army, go to college, establish a career with the New York State Labor Department—and contract a life-threatening illness at age thirty-five. I shall never forget the day: I was restless at the university where I was working on Long Island in late 1972. I kept thinking of "home" all day and finally at 4 P.M., I picked up the phone and called my sister Rosemary. "How did you know?" she asked me. "How did I know what?" I answered.

That day my brother Joe had been in the operating room since early morning as the doctors removed a thirty-inch spleen, and shortly after, considering the degree of malignancy, didn't want to take bets on how long he would live. Sometime after that, when I visited Joe, he told me he had this strange experience. He "saw" the inside of his body, and all through him were little bristles, like those on a brush.

This didn't make much sense until the lab reports were all back and Joe's doctor gave him the news. He had a fatal disease called Hairy Cell Leukemia, and the doctor, to explain to him what this meant, showed him what Joe had already "seen" in his strange and unexplainable visualization—"hairy" cells under the microscope.

Now commenced the battle, and Joe was determined to live despite the odds. It would be impossible to talk about the near-death times we, as a family, lived through with Joe. But there was a strong ray of hope in the doctor he eventually found—a hematologist by the name of Dr. Frank Lizzi, the most respected, at St. Peter's Hospital in Albany.

That was a familiar name to me and one day when I was visiting my brother in the hospital, I told him that when he was a tot, we had lived in a house on Irving Street where our landlord was name Lizzi.

Joe was aware of that. In fact, he said, our one-time landlord was the late grandfather of his Dr. Lizzi. It was like a light went on. Is it possible that his father was a shoemaker and his mother named Catuzza? Yes, said Joe.

They were his parents. Not only that, Dr. Lizzi was just three years younger than himself, my brother told me—as a realization hit both of us. Catuzza's baby, yet unborn, was to be the doctor who one day would save Joe's life! For Dr. Lizzi did just that, keeping him alive with every new drug and therapy that came along, until we got the miracle we prayed for—interferon, effective in the form of cancer Joe has, Hairy Cell Leukemia.

Last year, I watched Joe and Dr. Lizzi on television as they participated in a telethon for leukemia research. Side by side, they asked for dollars to keep the scientists working to make the discoveries that, as interferon had for Joe, will save lives.

What I saw for a moment was not two fine men in their early fifties. I saw a golden-haired child with his hand on the tummy of a somewhat blushing mother-to-be, and I marveled at the mystery of connections. Never would any of us have been able to imagine that the unborn baby would one day himself return that touch, carrying life with it.

And so, now, on Mother's Day, and many times between, I think of Catuzza—and say "thank you!"

Antoinette Bosco
Litchfield County Times

Love, Friendship and Miracles

The years teach much which the days never know.

Ralph Waldo Emerson

I have a very dear friend whom I have known for twenty-five years now. Debbie and I went to high school together, and even after I moved away, we kept in touch and visited each other whenever we could. She and I were close and shared something special that we did not realize until one summer. I was visiting her in Florida with my two children. She lived there with her husband of twenty years and their two cats. They seemed to have it all, but after three miscarriages, I was beginning to think maybe not everything. They were a wonderful and loving couple who wanted a child and deserved a child. That summer she broke down and told me of their recent loss, for the third time, and of the following testing, which showed that she was incapable of carrying a child. I didn't hesitate to offer myself to be a surrogate and said that I needed to run it by my husband. He was so supportive, and they were elated!

I started treatment at a fertility clinic near my Maryland home, and we began the hormone shots and patches to get us regulated and in sync. The big day came when I flew down to Florida for the implant. It was a very happy day for us all; even though I missed my daughter's birthday, I felt somehow that this was truly going to be another's "birthday" also. The days of waiting for the results were agonizing, but I felt sure it had worked. Why would these good people be denied something so precious? The call came from the doctor, and it was devastating to say the least. I didn't believe them at first; there must be a mistake—sometimes pregnancy tests were wrong! Why couldn't this work out for them? Maybe they were already as happy as any couple should be. Great home, great jobs, great family and friends, what more could they ask for? Maybe they were asking for too much? I just couldn't make sense of any of this.

During the months leading up to the procedure, I told only my teammate at school to explain my numerous absences, and afterwards I shared the experience with a very dear friend, Lori, who was like a little sister. A couple of months had passed when Lori came over for a visit. She said she was pregnant and decided to give the baby up for adoption. She was a single parent of one already, struggling financially, and this father was not taking responsibility for her present condition. She told me that she wanted my friends to have this baby, knowing what I did for them, she knew they were special people who would cherish this gift. It took some time for me to catch my breath, discuss this with her and call my friends. None of us could believe the chain of events . . . the circle of friendships. No wonder why I was not able to have their baby; they were meant to help Lori.

They started proceedings in Florida, and I supported Lori up here in Maryland. It was so reassuring to know how certain she was that she had made the right decision. When her due date was a week away, I took her to the airport. Everything went smoothly right up to the birth, and I was the first one called when the baby arrived! A boy was born healthy and already blessed with an extended family of love. I don't think he'll ever know the impact he made on so many lives. Baby Derek is going to be a year old this July.

Debbie Graziano

Book of Dreams

A dream is a wish your heart makes.

Walt Disney

A full moon hung in the sky as Lorianne Clark climbed out of bed, too anxious to sleep. Tiptoeing to the kitchen, she opened her journal.

Dear Dream, she penned. *You'll be in our lives soon—if only we're granted a miracle tomorrow!*

Growing up in Niagara Falls, Ontario, Lorianne toted a doll named Ginger around wherever she went. And as a teen, she'd stop mothers pushing carriages to admire their little ones.

"What's your name?" she cooed to a curly-topped toddler one afternoon.

Her mother smiled. "Her name is Dream," she said. "Because after years of trying—and dreaming—she came to us."

I'd do anything to be a mommy, too, Lorianne thought, touched by the woman's story.

And Lorianne's dream never changed as she met and fell in love with Rich. So shortly after they said "I do," they began trying.

But after two years . . . nothing.

"It'll happen someday, right?" Lorianne asked her gynecologist.

Frowning at the chart which noted her irregular, painful periods, he suggested she undergo an exploratory laparoscopy—which revealed endometriosis, a condition in which tissue grows outside the uterus.

In surgery, doctors removed 80 percent of the tissue. But afterward, there was grim news.

"You have stage-three endometriosis," the doctor warned. "The tissue may grow back and block your fallopian tubes. Your chances of conceiving aren't good."

At first, his warning was so heartbreaking, Lorianne refused to believe it. Everywhere she looked, it seemed, were cruel reminders of what she might never have: babies in diaper commercials, her sister-in-law's pregnant belly . . .

"I can't stop trying, no matter what the odds," she wept to Rich.

But month after month, Lorianne doubled over with cramps. *I always assumed I could have a baby*, she wept silently. *And now, I feel betrayed—by my own body.*

But somehow, she knew, she had to find a way to hold on to hope. So she began keeping a journal.

Dear Dream, she scrawled one morning. *This book will hopefully be special to you someday . . .*

Finally, the doctor suggested in vitro fertilization. "But first you'll need another laparoscopy, because I'm sure the adhesions have returned," he said.

I'm in the hospital, Lorianne wrote the night of the procedure. *But I'll do whatever I have to, again and again, until I have you, Dream!*

But during the procedure, doctors found that Lorianne was now in stage-four endometriosis—and it was choking her fallopian tubes.

"You can go ahead with the in vitro if you want," her doctor told her. "But at this point, your chances of conceiving are slim to none."

"Then those are the chances I'll have to take," Lorianne replied.

And now, the night before the in vitro, she sat in her kitchen—and her thoughts drifted back to the woman with the curly-headed tot. She waited years for her miracle—but it came, Lorianne remembered. Lifting her pen, she wrote, *I'm still afraid to get my hopes up. We have to pray . . .*

So that's what Lorianne did as she and Rich drove to the clinic, where a fertility team harvested seven eggs, then mixed them with Rich's sperm. Of the six that grew into embryos, three were implanted in Lorianne's uterus, the other three frozen for a second try.

Please, God, Lorianne prayed each night. *Let our dream come true!*

A month later, her prayers were answered: "You'll be parents by Halloween," the nurse announced.

"Pinch me!" Lorianne sang as Rich called everyone they knew.

And on October 22, 1993, Dream Marie Clark—with a mop of black hair—was laid on her mommy's chest. "I love you, Dream," Lorianne choked as Rich embraced "his girls."

And though she was sleep-deprived and often had tapioca in her hair, Lorianne treasured every moment of her "Dream": dancing with the baby when she was restless with colic, cheering as she took her first steps. And when Dream began talking, the little girl cradled Ginger—the same doll that Lorianne had played with a generation before—and dreamed her own dream.

"I want a sister!" Dream cried.

Lorianne and Rich exchanged glances. They'd often imagined a sibling for Dream. *But we've already been given one miracle,* Lorianne thought. *Do we dare hope for another?*

Then, at her next checkup, Lorianne learned the endometriosis was likely spreading. "The only way to possibly stop it is a hysterectomy," the gynecologist told her.

Time's running out! Lorianne gulped. She and Rich crossed their fingers as the frozen embryos were thawed and implanted in her uterus. But this time, it didn't work.

Three of us will have to be enough, Lorianne told herself. And though it broke her heart, she gave away Dream's stroller and high chair.

Then, on Dream's first day of preschool, Lorianne had a checkup. "Last period?" the nurse asked, and Lorianne estimated, "End of July?"

"You're late," she replied. "Perhaps you're pregnant."

"That's impossible!" Lorianne blurted. But a pregnancy test showed that she was!

"God was listening to us," Rich beamed. "It's destiny!"

That night, Lorianne wrote in her journal: *Dear Dream and Destiny: Soon I'll have two angels. I can't wait!*

And neither could Destiny Anne: She came into the world two weeks early—just before Mother's Day. "What a gift!" Lorianne wept.

Today, Lorianne is often stopped by admiring young women as she pushes Destiny's stroller, Dream alongside her. "What are your names?" they ask.

"Dream," the five-year-old says. "And this is Destiny!"

"There's gotta be a story behind those names," the passersby inevitably say.

"You bet there is," Lorianne replies. Then, beaming, she shares the tale of how she was twice blessed, inspiring yet another person to believe in miracles.

Barbara Mackey
Excerpted from Woman's World

Sickest Baby in the ICU

Erik arrived on a clear, cold October dawn—eight pounds, two ounces, healthy and untroubled. My husband, Jim, and I took him home the next day. He ate and slept and settled in. On Halloween our three-year-old daughter, Katie, thought he smiled at her jack-o'-lantern.

Then on his one-week birthday, Erik would not wake up to nurse. When I changed his diaper, his skin flushed deep red. I called the doctor. Newborns are funny creatures, he told me. Erik is fine.

That night I dreamed a jack-o'-lantern overturned and set the hall rug on fire. Even awake I smelled scorched pumpkin. I reached for Erik in the bassinet beside our bed. I woke Jim, and we took Erik's temperature: 104°F.

On the drive to Boston Children's Hospital, Erik lay motionless on my lap. "Breathe, Erik," I cried, shaking him. I was terrified he would die in my arms.

In the emergency room, a nurse wrapped a tiny blood-pressure cuff around Erik's arm. The machine would not register. "It's probably broken," she said. "Let's get another." But the next machine didn't work, and neither did the one after that.

"Please get help!" Jim urged. A doctor came, bringing a

portable heart monitor. He glued electrodes to Erik's chest and triggered a switch. A number flashed on the digital display: 278—about two times the normal infant heart rate.

A cardiac team rushed in, three women and four men in blood-spattered scrubs. Erik slept as they carried him to a treatment room three doors down, but we heard his screams during a spinal tap and, later, when they tried to shock his racing heart.

Erik was half-awake when they brought him back to us. I started to cry when I had to hand him to one of the doctors: Was I giving him up forever?

They strapped Erik to a stretcher, loaded his monitors and IV pumps on a cart and disappeared into the elevator the way they had come, in a clatter of clogs and rolling wheels.

Soon Jim and I were told our son had acute myocarditis —a life-threatening inflammation of the heart muscle. In newborns like Erik, a Coxsackie virus often causes the condition. No drugs exist to treat the virus; about a third of the children who contract it die.

Dr. Edward Walsh, our cardiologist, and Dr. David Wessel, director of the intensive care unit, placed Erik on life support and administered drugs to boost his blood pressure, support the heart and slow his metabolism. None of these measures improved his condition.

For the first few days, Erik laid on a gurney, small and naked beneath a tangle of IV lines and electrical leads. The heart monitor above his head showed a hurried scribble of peaks and valleys. I stared, mesmerized, at the digital readout: 281, 262, 212, 289.

The second day blended into the third, the third into the fourth. Erik's racing heart never dropped below 200. Each day, he weakened. Then, on his sixth day in the ICU, Erik seemed a bit better. His heart rate and blood pressure stabilized. And on the seventh day, he tried to breathe on his own. That afternoon, Dr. Wessel told Jim and me, "I think Erik's winning. My prediction is in three years, he'll be playing soccer."

At eight o'clock, when the night nurse arrived, Erik lay dozing, unbothered by the buzzers and bells of a dozen machines. I watched as she kissed my son on the forehead. "He's looking good," she said.

I nodded. I, too, had grown used to Erik's blue-black feet and swollen lips, to stitches in his scalp and groin, even to the false, hissing breath of the respirator.

Still, I felt uneasy. "I'm going downstairs for a while," I told the nurse.

A heavy November rain pounded on the roof of the hospital chapel. I sat in a rear pew and tried to pray. In front of me a man wept, forehead pressed into his hands. I recognized him from the sixth-floor lounge. His five-year-old daughter had received a heart transplant. He turned and smiled at me through his tears.

Then the doors of the chapel swung open. A man stood silhouetted. "Things are very bad," I heard my husband say. "They want to see us."

We ran to the elevators at the end of the hall. On the ride up, I pressed my hand to my mouth so I wouldn't scream. *Dr. Walsh won't let us down,* I thought as he ushered us toward the parents' lounge. *He has been with us from the start, has gone many nights without sleep for our son.*

A "Do Not Disturb" sign was taped to the lounge door. "We can't go in there," I said, then realized the sign was meant to exclude everyone but us.

Dr. Walsh closed the door. "Erik went into cardiac arrest thirty minutes ago," he told us. "We've been unable to resuscitate him. I'm so sorry."

Jim and I sat holding hands, but I remember feeling separated from my body. I did not see Dr. Wessel race through the halls in a tuxedo, summoned by beeper from a dinner. Nor did I see Dr. Walsh return to the resuscitation team that, against all hope, still pumped Erik's heart. I just sat there—disbelieving.

At Erik's bedside, Dr. Wessel searched through yards of readout tapes, studying patterns, frantic for an answer. Finally, someone switched the heart monitor off, and in that moment Dr. Wessel called for a syringe. Perhaps, he reasoned, fluid had built up in the sac that surrounds the heart and compressed the beating. He slid the needle deep inside Erik's chest and pulled. Fluid flowed into the tube. Erik's heart heaved, then pumped.

Dr. Walsh returned fifteen minutes later to the parents' lounge. He was crying. "There's been a major change," he said. "It's incredible. Erik is alive."

I came back to my body. "Can we see him?" Jim asked. "We need to see him."

Dr. Walsh cleared his throat.

"There's something you should know," he said. "We're not getting any neurological response. There's a possibility of brain damage."

When Jim and I saw Erik in the hour after Dr. Wessel had saved his life, his chest was punctured and bloodied, his mouth open in what looked like a scream. But what frightened me most were his eyes—unblinking pupils dilated wide. I looked into those vacant eyes and felt horror. *He's worse than dead,* I thought. *He's ruined.*

Jim stepped out of the room, and I was alone with my son. The nurse had turned the lights down: only digital displays lit Erik's face. His ventilator hoses gurgled quietly. The monitor display blinked—134, 132, 133—steady, steady.

I thought of disconnecting the ventilator and pulling every IV line. I wanted to take Erik in my arms and let him die. I was convinced that he would only suffer, that he'd been terribly violated. But I couldn't do it. I wrapped his swollen fingers around my thumb and began to sing to him.

At that moment I knew Erik's life was on a course unchangeable by human hands. Understanding that, on that most terrible of nights, set me free.

Three mornings after his heart had stopped, Erik opened his eyes. I filled a basin with water and sponged him, wiping away bits of blood and adhesive. His skin felt rubbery, his muscles toneless.

He was moved from intensive care to a medical wing on November 23, a day shy of four weeks old. The effects of the virus had subsided, but not before consuming half the strength of his heart. What was left could keep him alive, but it wouldn't be enough for him to grow.

During the next three weeks, Erik returned slowly to himself. He smiled—first at Jim, me, then at anyone who looked his way. On December twelfth, Dr. Walsh removed his feeding tube. That night Erik nursed, staring into my eyes, as though remembering the brief time we'd had before he got sick. I felt elated; he was mine again.

Yet every day we struggled with the possibility of losing him, with loving and letting go. No one knew how long Erik would live. His doctors talked about a transplant.

The morning of Erik's discharge, Dr. Walsh took him for a sonogram. We waited in our son's room, listening for the sound of bassinet wheels on linoleum.

When they came, they came fast, the glass top of the bassinet rattling noisily. Dr. Walsh banged the door open. His face was flushed. "Eighty percent!" he shouted. "Eighty percent!" Erik's heart was functioning at eighty percent!

Jim unhooked Erik from his monitors and tossed him in the air. Nurses and residents crowded into the room. Someone brought balloons and cake. We turned music on and had a party.

The doctors called it a miracle, and it was. I think of that when Erik snuggles against me in the morning, when he races his cars across the floor, when he rides with Katie on her two-seat tricycle. I think of the miracle most at night, when I rock him and sing, and he sings, too.

Twice a year we return to see Dr. Walsh. Everyone at Boston Children's Hospital knows Erik as one of the sickest babies ever to leave the ICU. A crowd gathers to watch him play blocks in the playroom.

Today Erik is four. He is quick to laugh and slow to cry. He is naughtier than his sister is. He floats sneakers in the toilet and scribbles in books. He loves Big Bird and bulldozers and hates baths.

There are no signs of brain damage. His heart strength is at 90 percent. Outside the hospital Erik looks like any other child. At the park where he plays, he usually runs for the swings, but sometimes a mud puddle catches his eye. He stomps and splashes. Water sloshes over his boot tops; bits of mud dot his face. He looks like any other child, but I know he is a miracle.

Cindy Anderson

7

MEMORABLE MOMENTS

The happiest moments of my life have been the few which I have passed at home in the bosom of my family.

Thomas Jefferson

Generations

Cradling my pregnant stomach, I plop down on the cushioned porch swing like a sack of potatoes, and elevate my swollen feet on the armrest. I relax and feel the summer heat mix with the cooler air of upcoming twilight. It is peaceful in the country. It has been a fun but tiring day at our annual family reunion, filled with tons of food and multiple verses of "You Are My Sunshine." Eating and singing are the two things my family does best, or at least with the most zeal.

Only my grandmother and I are left back at the house. The rest of the family opted to go to the movies. Hearing the sound of clinking glass, I gaze up from my comfortable nest into the kitchen window. I study the aging profile of my grandmother. Seventy-five years old, full of arthritis, yet proud, she still will not let anyone else do her dishes. She is the hardest worker I know, always tending to everyone's needs before her own.

I used to try to change her selflessness. I remember a conversation when I attempted to open her eyes to equal rights. "Really, Grandma, you never do anything for yourself. Now that Grandpap is retired, it would only be fair that he help out with the household chores."

"But I enjoy my routine," she had responded, confused by my frustration. "Besides, I like to keep busy; it keeps me young."

"You could at least get a dishwasher," I had encouraged.

"If I had a dishwasher, what in the world would I do after dinner?" After that conversation I stopped trying to enlighten her to the nineties.

Taking in a deep breath, I continue to drift back in time to my childhood memories of the summers I spent at my grandparents' house. After dinner, my grandmother and I would sit on the porch swing and needlepoint. The rainbow colors of thread mesmerized me. I would line them up like a big rainbow and try to fit every color into my stitching. That was over fifteen years ago, before arthritis attacked her fingers, making her hobby too painful to pursue after a long day.

I hear the water turn off in the kitchen, and then the voice of my grandmother calling through the screen. "I think I'll let these dishes air dry. That'll give us more time together before the others get back. Give me a minute to change into my housecoat. Okay, Mom?"

Mom? I am confused for a moment until I realize she is referring to me. "Sounds good," I answer proudly, my heart skipping a beat as I feel my first step toward membership in the motherhood club.

My grandmother returns in her worn flowered housecoat. "Here," she smiles, handing me a present. "This is for the baby."

I open the package and look inside. Raggedy Ann and Andy dolls stare back at me from perfectly embroidered faces, just like the ones she handmade for me twenty-five years ago. Speechless, I look at Grandmother with tears in my eyes, comprehending the pain she endured in her hands to make the dolls.

"I've made every grandchild a set of Raggedy dolls. I'm

not about to stop now," she explains directly to my belly.

I never felt closer to my grandmother. The little human being growing inside me bridged our generation gap. I have a new respect for her. Before now, I never gave her much credit as a role model for today's woman. As it turns out, I was looking in the wrong places.

Sherrie Page Najarian

I Was Chosen

It was time for bed and I really didn't mind too much. It meant Mommy would smooth my sheets and crawl in my bed with me. I'd snuggle in her arms and she'd rub my hair and tell me how much she loved me. If it wasn't too late and Mommy wasn't too tired, I might get to hear The Story before we said our prayers together.

I never grew tired of hearing her tell The Story. It was so special because it was about me. Mommy would begin by saying, "Your daddy and I always wanted a baby. We wanted one for so long, and we kept praying that I would get pregnant and have a baby. But after several years when I didn't get pregnant, we began to realize that God had something even better for us. He decided that he was going to give us a very special baby—a baby that another lady was not able to take care of. He wanted parents who would be just right for this very special baby. Guess who that very special baby was? You!"

"Mommy, tell me about the day you got me."

"Well, Tucker," she would continue, "That was the most exciting day in my life! It began when the telephone rang, and a voice on the other end said, 'Mrs. Freeman, your beautiful baby girl has just been born. Would you like to come see her?'

"I called your daddy at the office and he raced home and got me and we hurried to the hospital. At first we stood outside the window where all the new babies were and just looked at them, trying to figure out which one was you! When we got to the end of the row you turned your head and looked at us and seemed to smile!

"We couldn't wait to take you home and introduce you to our family and friends. When we drove up to the house, there were lots of friends who had come to bring you presents! You have always been such a gift to us. Why, the smartest thing Daddy and I ever did in our lives was adopt you!"

Each time Mother told me The Story she got excited. She never tired of telling it, and I never got tired of hearing her tell it. From the beginning she made me feel that being adopted was tremendously special, that I had somehow been chosen.

When I was about seven months pregnant with my own child, my mother came to visit. It was one of those really uncomfortable days, and the baby was kicking me non-stop. As I groaned and held my stomach, my mother said, "It must be amazing to feel her kick."

Suddenly, it dawned on me that my mother had never felt a baby inside her womb.

"Mother," I said, "come and put your hands on my stomach. I want you to feel your grandchild."

The look of awe on my mother's face as she felt her granddaughter kick in the womb was so precious for me. I realized that I was able to give my mother a gift she had not been able to experience personally. She had given me so many gifts and finally I was able to share a very personal one with her.

Tucker Viccellio as told to Susan Alexander Yates and
Allison Yates Gaskins

THE FAMILY CIRCUS By Bil Keane

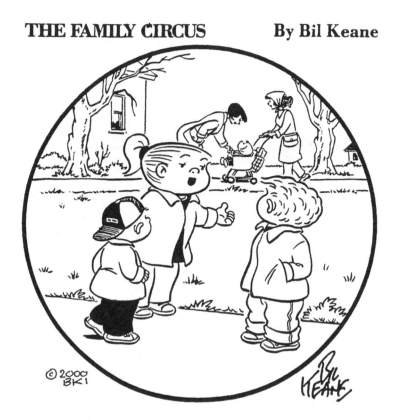

"We came from Mommy's tummy.
But Joseph is adopted, so he came from
his mommy's heart."

Keeping the High Watch

Almost home, fifteen minutes ahead of schedule, I had just enough time to change clothes before jumping back into the car for a forty-five mile commute to meet a real estate agent who was showing me a property in my soon-to-be "new neighborhood." As luck would have it, I got stuck at the longest stoplight in the area.

While waiting for the light to change, I caught a glimpse of a rather large low-flying bird. A very small bird appeared to be nipping at the large bird's tail, as if in attack. But after watching awhile, I realized that the larger bird was the mother and surmised that the small bird was her offspring taking its fledgling flight. Suddenly, the baby bird lost altitude and fluttered erratically, obviously unable to stay aloft. The mother swooped down and lifted the baby on her back into the windless clear-blue sky, and then pulled away again. The baby awkwardly regained its flying ability with the mother only inches away. Slowly the mother moved a few feet to the side, and then a few feet below. Baby was doing just fine.

I was so mesmerized, I didn't notice that the light had turned green until the cars behind me started honking their horns. I drove slowly, observing my birds. Watching this momentous occasion for baby and the loving, protective measures by its mother had suddenly become more important than any scheduled appointment. So it would delay my meeting fifteen more minutes. This was life!

I thought back to when my baby took her first steps. Initially I held her hands and then, ever so gently, I released my grip, but kept my hands close enough to catch her if necessary. My eyes swelled with tears. I felt such love for this mother bird who nurtures and was now helping to release her baby to follow its own life path. I thought again of my daughter, now grown with a nine-month-old baby of her own, experiencing these same kinds of poignant moments that only a mother can understand.

We release our young so many times, in so many ways: we help them take their first steps; send them off to school; watch as they go on their first dates; wish them well as they go away to college; and give them away in marriage. But we never release them from our hearts.

Mom and baby bird were soaring freely as I approached my garage. Now with no time to spare—I raced for the door. The phone began to ring. My first inclination was to let the machine answer it, but I somehow felt compelled to pick up. *Another five minutes down the drain,* I thought.

My daughter was calling from her home, fifteen hundred miles away, with news that her son, my grandson, had minutes earlier just taken his firsts steps. I began to cry. I believed that I had been there in some beautiful, unexplainable way, God had shared the moment with me.

I called my real estate agent and had her rearrange the appointment for a few hours later that day. I went for a walk on the beach and sat awhile, just gazing at the horizon. Talking a deep breath, I looked up. Birds soared overhead, and my grandson had started his journey through life. Carefully, I hoped, one step at a time.

Eileen Davis

Grandpa's Surprise

My husband has a rather portly build, with a sizable potbelly.

When our daughter was expecting her second child, my husband and I went to her house to take care of her three-year-old girl.

The first night, our little granddaughter made the rounds to kiss us all goodnight. After she kissed her mother's cheek, she then kissed her mother's tummy, bidding the unborn baby goodnight.

She ran down the hall to bed, then suddenly ran back to the living room, stopping in front of her grandfather. She bent over, kissed his belly and announced, "I forgot to kiss Grandpa's baby goodnight!"

Ruth M. Henshaw

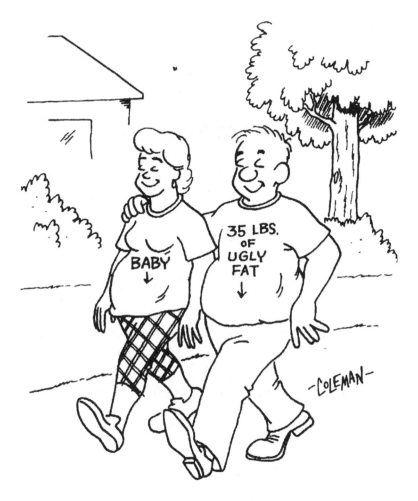

Reprinted by permission of Ronald Coleman. ©2000 Ronald Coleman.
Coleman@cartoonfactory.com

Love Notes

One sunny afternoon in May, when pink azalea, purple wisteria, and white dogwood painted our backyard in vibrant colors any child would love, my husband, Allen, called to tell me that finally a baby might be available for us to adopt.

We wasted no time contacting the attorney handling the case. We quickly discovered the deadline was *now*. The birth mother would collect the applications that afternoon. With the clock ticking, I answered the questions about why we would make good parents.

Several weeks went by, with no word.

One rainy afternoon at the post office, I saw Cindy, who worked with the attorney. I asked, "Have you heard anything?"

With downcast eyes, she answered, "I'm sorry. The birth mother picked up the applications, but she has disappeared."

Disappointed, I relayed the news to Allen.

Over the months ahead, I pondered what might have been and wondered about the birth mother.

In December, I received an unexpected phone call from

Cindy. She exclaimed, "The girl is back in town, and she has selected you and Allen!"

Our lives had never been more chaotic. We both had full-time careers and Allen had added the extra duties of becoming mayor of our town. Still, we were thrilled about the "possibility" even though we were warned over and over not to get our hopes up. But how could we not?

So the countdown began.

At once I wanted to order nursery wallpaper, until Allen pleaded, "Please, Debbie, no decorating and no baby shower. You'll be too disappointed if it doesn't work out." Instead we took care of the financial and medical arrangements. A social worker inspected our home—and us. There were mandatory physicals, including checkups for venereal diseases.

This last experience led me to ask our attorney to obtain a family health history from the birth mother. The request resulted in a series of notes that bounced back and forth on index cards between the mother and me. Eventually our correspondence shifted away from discussions of health. She asked, "What do you consider a happy home? A good education? Appropriate discipline?

Little by little, I began to think like a mother. Together we were preparing for the birth of the baby—hers and mine.

And oddly enough, this stranger turned into a friend.

Though neither of us wanted to meet, our notes revealed that we shared similar interests, such as the theater, walking on the beach and reading. Even our printing looked identical. I also discovered that she was articulate, humorous, mature and selfless in her desire to provide a loving family for her baby.

One cold February day, I received a jubilant call from Cindy. She said, "Congratulations, you have a baby girl!"

"Is she okay? How is the mother?" I was ecstatic. "They

are both fine—just fine," Cindy said, laughing.

Tears streamed down my face, I called Allen. I could barely get the words out. "We have a baby girl."

Within hours word of the baby spread through our small town. Friends loaned us a car seat and a cradle. Onlookers watched as we raced from store to store piling our buggy high with pink diapers, tiny smocked dresses, sleepers and pastel blankets.

Meanwhile, the birth mother held the baby, making sure she was healthy. She was adamant that no one adopt her but us.

"This little piggy went to the market," I said as Allen laughed. "And her nose looks like yours," I said. In fact, our baby *did* look like him.

As I dug into the hospital's gift bag, I saw the final letter from my friend, tucked beneath the baby wipes and the lotion. I wasn't able to open it just yet.

Falling in love with the baby came naturally. But I did not expect to feel love for a stranger when Allen and I decided to adopt; and I did—I came to love the birth mother. Thankfully she would always be our bond.

So with tears flowing, I read her love-filled note, which ended, "I gave her life, now you give her love." My note back would have said, "We always will!"

Debra Ayers Brown

To Our Baby Girl

We both love you, and
We both have hopes and dreams for your future.

She carried you in her body for nine months;
I carried you in my dreams for five years.

She labored through birth;
I labored through INS, social workers and foreign law.

She is nature;
I am nurture.

She wonders if are you healthy;
I sit and rock you wondering when your fever will go
   down.

She wonders if you have enough to eat;
I wonder should I make you eat your broccoli.

She wonders if are you happy;
I love to hear you laugh.

She wonders if are you loved;
My heart melts with every smile and breaks with every
  tear I soothe.

She wonders what you look like;
I proudly display your pictures all over the house.

She hopes you get a good education;
I sit and help you with your homework every night.

She wonders what you will grow up to be like;
I teach you to be strong, independent and to believe in
  yourself.

She wonders if you will marry and have children;
I help you plan your wedding day and cry when I hold
  my grandchild for the first time.

She gave you life;
I am grateful to her every day that you are a part of my life.

She will always wonder about you;
I will always be thankful to her for bringing you into this
  world.

She will always be your biological mother;
I will always be Mommy.

Audrie LaVigne

Baby Toys

My gynecologist was seeing a pregnant patient who had brought along her young daughter to the appointment. The young girl had brought along numerous toys, and as the mother hopped up on the exam table, the gynecologist made conversation with the youngster.

"My you have a lot of nice toys there," he said.

"I brought them for the baby," she replied.

With a puzzled look the gynecologist said, "Well, how is the baby going to play with them now?"

The girl replied, "I thought while we were here, you could put them in there for me!"

Lynne Murphy

A Friendly Face

It was the beginning of November. I was larger—"larger than life!"—my husband, Jeff told me. I had a belly the size of three basketballs. I was expecting our first child and I was scared to death. It was just my husband and me; no family no close friends to share in our excitement, our terror. We were stationed in Japan and had lived there for two years when I became pregnant.

When I noticed the first pangs of labor, my husband and I raced through the crowded streets of Japan. Okay, raced isn't quite the right word. It was more like "turtled" through the streets of Japan. Our hospital was at Yokota Air Force Base, which was only thirty miles away, but usually took us two hours to get to. I was too scared to notice the woman he nearly hit, the dog he almost ran over and the shopping cart he swerved around, and too tired to care. I did notice that he managed to hit every red light and a few train crossings.

Finally we got through the gates of the base and to the hospital. My contractions had subsided so the hospital told us to return home and rest. It was a false alarm. As we left, I noticed a rather tall woman, very much with child, being admitted to the delivery ward. We smiled in passing and I headed out the doors.

I cried a lot on the way home. I was so scared and dreaded another drive to the hospital. But what really upset me was that I was going to have a baby, and I had no one else to share it with. I was lucky to have my husband there. His squadron had deployed on a four-month cruise two weeks earlier. The commander allowed Jeff to stay behind until our child was born, then he had to meet up with the ship. That upset me too, that my husband would miss the first four months of his first child's life; that I would be a single mom and have to deal with not only my own recovery, but also learn how to care for an infant.

"If only I had my mom! Or your mom! Or some close friends!" I sobbed to my husband. He felt terrible, but there was little he could do.

That night, the pains started again and grew in frequency. I kicked my husband awake and told him it was time to go. This time it was three in the morning. There was little traffic and we made it to the hospital in record time.

Sixteen hours and a difficult delivery later, I gave birth to a boy we named Eric. We were shocked, because the Japanese doctor who gave me an ultrasound a few months before said he was sure it was a girl. At least, we thought he said girl. While everything we bought was feminine, frilly and pink, we were thrilled that our Emma was really an Eric.

I was wheeled into my room, which I had to share with another new mother, and Eric was whisked away to the nursery. There was a curtain separating me from the other mother but I could hear voices and the quiet gurgles of a newborn. I lay staring at Jeff.

"Can you believe we have a little boy?" he asked all smiles. I smiled and nodded. Then the tears came to my eyes.

"What's the matter?" Jeff sat down beside me.

"I'm supposed to be happy. Our parents should be here to meet their first grandchild. Our brothers and sisters and best friends should be here." I felt my chin quiver.

"They'll see him soon," Jeff said. He bent over and kissed my forehead. "Should I call home?" he asked.

"Sure," I let out a big yawn. I couldn't move. My body ached. I felt like a Mack truck had hit me. And worse, the nurse would be in soon to get me up and to the bathroom. "They'll be surprised to know we had a boy."

Jeff picked up the phone. "What's your parents' number?"

I gave him the number and he called home to tell everyone we had a baby boy. After he hung up I heard a voice from behind the curtain.

"Excuse me," said someone quietly.

My husband drew back the curtain and we looked at the tall woman I had seen earlier at the hospital.

"I heard you calling home and recognized the area code," she started. "Are you from Massachusetts?"

"My wife is," said Jeff pointing at me.

"Where in Mass?" asked the woman.

"Oh, it's a real small town between Boston and Cape Cod," I said.

"You probably don't know it."

"What's the name?"

"Norwell," I said.

The woman's eyes lit up and her jaw dropped.

"I'm from Norwell, too!"

I looked at her, my eyebrows scrunched tight. I didn't recognize her.

"What's your name?"

She told me and I immediately gave her mine. We stared at each other in disbelief.

"You're Kelly from South Street?" I asked. I sat up in my bed and straightened my hair.

"Yep. Can you believe this?" She was holding a small bundle and rocking her arms back and forth.

"This is amazing," I said. Jeff and Kelly's husband shook hands. I had known Kelly since elementary school. We went through high school together until she moved away some time around our senior year. We didn't hang out together but had the same homeroom and many classes together. Now, ten years later we were having babies together on the other side of the world. She had grown quite tall since I knew her and her hair was different. But when she told me her name I immediately recognized her. Our babies were due on the same day, but both decided to come late. Kelly had given birth to a beautiful baby girl named Samantha.

The remainder of our time in the hospital was spent going through yearbooks, which our husbands dug up for us. We gave interviews to the base newspapers. No one could believe that two high school friends would be reunited in the delivery ward of a military hospital, half way around the world.

My prayers were answered, too. At the moment Kelly spoke up, I was completely exhausted and filled with such sadness, longing for a familiar face from home.

While my husband was shipped off two weeks later, Kelly and I kept in contact. Every Christmas I receive a card from her and Samantha, letting me know how they are doing.

Jennifer Reed

Unexpected Blessings

When the adoption agency said we were matched for a baby boy, we were overjoyed. We hugged and kissed in celebration that our dream was about to come true. So when the counselor said we should be ready to fly to the opposite coast for his due date on April 27, just over a week away, we didn't hesitate for a second in saying we would be there.

Most expectant mothers have nine months to prepare—we had just nine days. We had been expecting a full two-year wait for a child. We were shocked when the call came just three months after we completed the paperwork. "Is the nursery ready?" asked a business associate. Well, not exactly. In fact, we had nothing for a baby. The would-be nursery in our 1840s fixer-upper farmhouse was water damaged and very badly in need of rewiring as well as new walls, a new ceiling and floor. Once the room was finished, we could begin purchasing items for our future addition to the family.

Nine days? We could do it! After all, it's not every day that a couple can fulfill their dream of bringing a baby into their lives.

We worked during the day and worked like mad by

night. The thought of finally having a child of our own kept us going. As the baby's due date neared, we were almost finished restoring the room. We made a whirlwind trip through two stores to buy the basic necessities—a diaper bag, diapers, baby wipes and blankets. Friends, family and sometimes even complete strangers who had heard our story showed up with used baby furniture, clothes and a host of other necessities to help us be ready in time.

As we boarded the flight with a stocked diaper bag and borrowed car seat in hand, we had accomplished nearly all of our goals—except for painting and putting up the last of the wood trim work in the nursery. The baby's room would not be exactly as we had pictured it, but somehow we thought our son would not notice if a few final touches came later.

Three weeks and a long airplane ride later, my husband and I walked through the door of our home with our new son. The moment was one of indescribable joy for us. As we put our son to sleep in his cousin's crib, we noticed an unexpected surprise: the painting was completed and the trim work placed! The nursery was finished! Next, we noticed that the refrigerator had been stocked with several meals for us.

Friends and family came throughout the next few days to see our new son and continued to bring items we needed, such as a playpen and a highchair. When our son went through a bout of colic, my mother-in-law gave us one of the best gifts of all—the opportunity to get some precious sleep.

Reflecting on our first few hours home as a family, we now realize that our blessings extended far beyond our new son. Little did we realize, we had already been part of a caring extended family, larger than we could have ever imagined.

Cynthia Hummel

Man in Labor

I think my oldest son thought he'd just stay as snug as a bug in a rug for as long as he could while I was carrying him toward the end of my pregnancy.

The doctor decided to induce labor after I had gone a couple of weeks past the due date. I was told to walk the halls at the hospital so the baby would drop a little into the birth canal and labor pains would begin.

My husband and I walked all afternoon and for almost three hours into the evening and nothing happened. We decided to go back into the labor room and sit down and relax a while.

While there, my husband decided to find a bathroom. I suggested that he use the one attached to the labor room because I was the only woman in labor that evening.

Within seconds, a couple of nurses burst into the room, flew by me and quickly opened the bathroom door.

There stood my husband—taking care of business! More embarrassed than I ever saw him before, he muttered, "I pushed the emergency button by mistake." (Instead of the light switch!) He grabbed the doorknob and quickly shut the door.

The nurses burst out laughing, and I did, too.

I laughed so hard, I laughed myself into labor pains!

Very shortly, our healthy beautiful son was born. And while my husband and I rejoiced over our precious newborn, the nurses continued to recount their highlight of the day—the very first man in labor!

Brenda Ford Miller

The Decision

Not all mothers are blissfully happy when their first child is born. For some, the circumstances are difficult and confusing. That was the case the night my girlfriend dropped me off at St. Anthony's Hospital. Alone and afraid, I was taken to a small room and told to put on a gown and lie on the bed. The nurses didn't speak much to me—I was unmarried, young, alone, and pregnant, and such a thing was frowned upon, especially in the South in the early 1970s. Alone I bore the heaviness of the labor of childbirth in a darkened labor room, only occasionally checked by nurses who didn't show much compassion.

Little did I know of the workings of such a place—of what had already been planned for me. The hospital had a social service director, and when an unmarried, teenage girl came in to give birth, they had a deserving family already in mind for the new child. They would help me see how inadequate and unprepared I was for childbirth, much less parenthood. And of course they were right.

After my delivery, I woke from a deep sleep. In the dark hours before dawn, I looked around the room: old linoleum yellowed on the floor beneath my railed bed; one small light on the wall behind me; a metal chair against the wall. *Where was my baby? Was it a girl, a boy?*

I cried out, and in my drug-induced state, I vaguely remembered my mother bending over me. "It's a girl," she whispered. "She is healthy and beautiful."

When I awoke some hours later I rang for the nurse and asked for my baby. She seemed puzzled, but after much persistence on my part, she brought in a small bundle and laid her in my arms. The baby was so beautiful, so small, so perfect. Thick, dark, curly hair topped her round pink face. Her eyes were as dark as raisins and her skin was as smooth as the finest silk. A baby! A little person! My mind was swirling with thoughts and my heart overflowing with emotions. I had no idea what I was doing, but this I did know: My life would never be the same.

Soon after, a social worker came to visit me. She explained that they had a family, a special and loving family who had been waiting for so long for a child they could love and care for. She talked to me about responsibility, my future, and the opportunities I would lose trying to raise a baby alone. Much of what she said was true. I was so young—only sixteen years old—but I felt deep in my soul that this was the most important decision I would perhaps ever make.

I told her I would pray. I didn't know much about prayer—I had been to church as a young girl with my grandmother and my mother, but I had no deep religious feelings of my own. There had certainly been times when I had prayed in the past, "Please get me out of this mess!" but I knew this was a different kind of prayer. I needed an answer. I waited for it. I listened. Day after day I listened, with the socialworker encouraging me to do the right thing for this little girl. Each afternoon, friends visited me, quiet about their opinions. Each evening my mother and grandmother visited, also quiet. Everyone was waiting for me. I was waiting for God.

After nine days the pressure was mounting. The hospital wanted my bed. The social services department wanted my baby. I wanted my answer. One afternoon my girlfriend tiptoed into my room. She sat on the side of my bed and took my hand in hers. Eyes brimming with tears, she shared her hidden secret with me. She, too, had been an unwed teenage mother. She, too, had faced this decision. She, too, had been afraid. In heart-breaking detail she described her feelings and concerns at the time. She knew exactly how I was feeling! She told me that now, at age twenty-one, she knew in her heart that letting go of her baby to a loving and wonderful family had been the right thing to do, and she encouraged me to do the same. She left, and I was alone with my thoughts. I had prayed for God to give me an answer. Was this it? Logically it made sense. It must be right, but what was wrong with my heart? It felt like it was breaking.

That night my mother came again to see me. She had kept her opinions to herself as I had struggled over the past few days, waiting for an answer to my prayers. She knew more, saw more, felt more than she shared with me. It would be many years later when she would confirm the events of that night with me.

I had been waiting for her to come. All afternoon I'd cried. I told my mother of the visit with my friend, of the story she had shared. I told her that after talking to my friend I had decided to let my baby go home with the family that waited for her. I had decided in my mind, but what was I going to do about my heart? The feelings there were quite different. I felt as if I was grieving. I felt something had died inside of me.

At last, my mother began to share her feelings with me. She did not agree with my girlfriend and told me of her own impressions over the past several days. I don't remember much of what she said, for I was listening— listening to the sound of my baby crying in the nursery. I got up and walked down the corridor to the baby nursery at the end of a long hall. It didn't occur to me that it would have been impossible for me to hear a baby crying so far away and in an enclosed room, much less to distinguish the sound of my own crying child. But somehow I just knew she was crying and that I needed to go to her.

I was unaware of my mother following me down the hall to the nursery—I was conscious only of the sound of my daughter's cry. Then something happened that even now is almost too miraculous to describe.

As I peered through the glass wall that separated me from my crying child, a bright, white light seemed to descend from the ceiling above her and encompassed the crib in which she lay. It was luminous and shone directly on her little body. Then I heard these words, as clearly as if someone were speaking in my ear. "This is your child. She was sent here to you. No one will ever be able to love her as you will." Suddenly, joy swelled within my heart and peace filled my aching soul, and I knew God had truly heard and answered my prayers. The next morning, a long ten days after her birth, I took my precious daughter home with me.

The years that followed were certainly not easy. I worked as a waitress, spent two years in college, and made many mistakes along the way. I know the decision to keep the baby would not be right for many young women; giving up a baby for adoption is a noble act of love. And yet time after time, the voice I heard and the light I saw that night gave me the courage to know I had done the right thing for this particular baby.

I had been given a clear understanding that this child would need *my* love and devotion in her life. But what soon became even more evident was that I would need *her* love and support to carry me through some difficult years. That daughter has now graduated from college and is making a wonderful life on her own. I cannot imagine what my life would have been without her.

Cindy Barksdale

Fingerprints

From our first date during our senior year of high school, through college graduation, fourteen years of marriage, and the births of four children, my husband and I have been inseparable. Two against the world. We leaned on each other for support and backed each other's decisions. Until the summer of 1997.

That summer I began to feel a tug on my heart in an unexpected direction. I'd been aware for awhile of the many little girls orphaned in China due to China's one-child policy. My heart was drawn to their plight and filled with a desire to do something for at least one child. This desire intensified when our "baby" turned three years old. Our children were growing up so quickly!

And we had been so blessed—first of all to be born in the United States where material things abound and freedom is taken for granted. We had a strong marriage, a healthy family, good jobs and a nice home. We also had an empty bedroom, fully stocked with every item of baby paraphernalia known to man. To me it was an obvious decision. We were the perfect family to adopt a child.

I broached the idea to my husband, hoping it would be

as obvious to him as it had been to me. After all, we loved kids. We'd admired the beauty of Asian children for years. We'd even joked about "when we adopt our little girl from China." And I knew he was also aware of how blessed we are.

"Are you crazy?" His vehement rejection of my idea shocked me. "Don't you think four kids is enough? Besides, we don't have that kind of money!"

No reassurances on my part convinced him one iota. He honestly thought I had a screw loose. I repeatedly tried to explain my logic to him. But time and again over the next weeks, he countered with all the reasons we shouldn't adopt. The rift caused us both tremendous pain. In the past, when we'd disagreed, we'd always been able to find some middle ground. But this time there was no such thing. You can't adopt half a child.

When all my logic got me nowhere, feeling utterly helpless, I began to pray. Not only for the baby who by this time seemed alive in my heart, but for unity between us. As much as I longed for a child on the other side of the world, I wanted a stable marriage even more. If adoption was really the right path for our family, then a power higher than my own was going to have to notify John. And so far there was no sign of that happening.

Depression compounded by guilt filled my days. Guilt because I knew I should be content with the four little blessings that I had already. I carried on for their sakes, comforted by the daily routines of meals and laundry, hugs and squabble arbitration, yet haunted by the conviction that we should be doing more in this world.

I knew that to do right by another child, my husband would have to enter into parenting wholeheartedly, and not just to please me. That seemed an impossible dream. But I had heard stories of other couples who had resolved similar dilemmas. I decided to pray and leave him alone to mull things over. My naturally optimistic nature watched hopefully for any slight sign of change.

Many times during those long slow months, I wondered if I was crazy to be nurturing such a dream. Yet every time I resolved to give it up, God placed another reminder in our path. Once it was a TV documentary about China. Another time a beautiful Asian couple in a restaurant. Another time a busload of Asian teenagers swarming onto an usually quiet beach.

It seemed adoption was not meant to fade from our minds. So I waited. Prayed, fiercely at times: "Remember all those motherless babies over there, Lord. Remember my arms that ache for another child. Remember us." And finally, after an endlessly long wait, a miracle began to happen. My husband began to ask questions about adoption. Barely daring to breathe, I'd answer, affecting a nonchalance that I was far from feeling. I'd mull over each casual question for days, afraid that I'd attached too much significance to it.

But then another question would come. And another. As we talked, he shared his fears over adopting from China—the paperwork, the two-week stay in a foreign country, the possible special needs of the child. We began to discuss Korea—the adoption process is simpler there—less paperwork, a shorter wait, no travel requirement. The conversations were cautious, theoretical—leaving me simultaneously jubilant and riddled with uncertainty. Could he really be seriously considering it?

Christmas was approaching, and my husband's mood still seemed miraculously favorable. When he asked me what I wanted for Christmas, I told him all I wanted was his fingerprints—for the criminal background check, the first step in the adoption process. To my surprise, he didn't seem angry at my request. In the following weeks, he dropped hints that made me hope for a wonderful Christmas surprise.

And yet there were worrisome moments too, the normal kind of moments all parents have, with kids fighting, or vomiting or hunting lost shoes. At times like that, he would turn to me in a huff, "We don't need another kid!"

"No," I would say, "but a child out there needs us."

Several times during December he asked me to expand my Christmas list, probably hoping I would request a Crock-Pot or a computer instead of a child. I staunchly insisted that his fingerprints were all I wanted.

By the time Christmas Eve came, I could hardly stand the suspense. I vowed to graciously accept his decision, whatever it might be, but my stomach was all in knots.

In the midst of the chaos of four kids ripping gifts open as fast as they could, John casually tossed a tiny gift my way. With trembling fingers I opened it. Inside was a little gold key chain with a coin-shaped gold medallion on it that said, "God Keeps His Promises."

It was a sweet little thing, and I forced enthusiasm into my voice to thank John, thinking maybe I'd pinned my hopes on something too big. My heart felt so fragile and fearful. Maybe all the hints of the previous weeks were just a fabrication of my hopeful heart. I tried to remind myself what an enormous thing I was asking of him. Maybe that dream-child from far away was not meant for our family.

But John was still watching me. Finally he said, "What's on the back of the key chain?"

Heart thudding, I flipped the medallion over.

There, etched in the smooth gold on the back of the medallion, was a single golden thumbprint.

Mary Ostyn

Baby for Sale

When I took my baby daughter to the supermarket for the first time, I dressed her in pink from head to toe. At the store, I placed her in the shopping cart, put my purchases around her and headed for the checkout line.

A small boy and his mother were ahead of me. The child was crying and begging for some special treat. *He wants some candy or gum and his mother won't let him have any,* I thought.

Then I heard his mother's reply. "No!" she said, looking in my direction. "You may not have a baby sister today. They don't have any more. That lady got the last one!"

Marsha Priesmeyer

For Now

On Mother's Day I will have been a mother for exactly seven months. So I guess that makes me a New Mother— one of those starry-eyed creatures still overwhelmed by wonder at the miracle she produced.

I have several friends who are Old Mothers. They say things like: "Hope yours isn't a whiner. Just wait till she's a teenager. Better enjoy her while you can; she'll be grown before you know it."

I may make many mistakes in my life, but neglecting to enjoy my baby will not be among them. For now, she is all promise and all potential. And for a little while, she is all mine.

The day may come when I am horrified at what she chooses to wear on a date, but for now, she wears pink things with Zwieback crumbs and she giggles when I put on her undershirt.

She may someday find it embarrassing to be seen with me in public, but for now, she stares up at me from the grocery cart and reaches for me when people coo at her in the checkout line.

She may rush off to school one day without saying good-bye, but for now, her whole body wiggles with delight when I come into the room the first thing each day.

One day she will grow up and go on her own way, and that is how it should be. But for now, after a bath and bottle, I can cradle her all downy and drowsy against my neck. I breathe deeply of her sweet-soft baby smell and I exult in it, and will remember it—always.

Caroline Castle Hicks

Love in the Rearview Mirror

I found love in the rearview mirror.

Over the weekend, my wife, the boys and I were running errands in the minivan. But neither Jeremy nor Matthew had slept well the night before so they were exhausted.

During the ride, Matthew's head started to bob as he fought to keep his eyes open. Soon, though, he fell asleep and his head dropped to the left, next to Jeremy.

At the same time, Jeremy, who was almost asleep himself, saw his brother sleeping and moved to the right to support Matthew's head with his shoulder. And, in a moment that will never leave me, he turned and gently kissed the top of Matthew's head, not knowing I was watching.

And, that's where I began to worry. Because I knew that no matter how hard I tried, no matter what I wrote, I would never be able to capture that sacred, perfect moment when my sons became something else, something deeper than what we know. Something that sits quietly behind what we see waiting patiently for us to discover it. Something that can be found in awkward first kisses, mothers rocking their newborn babies, husbands whispering their wives' names, and the quiet moments of courage and caring that happen all around and within us.

But, no matter how much I worry, I can't stop searching for the words. Because love wouldn't have it any other way.

Jim Warda

Breathe

Since I am an actively working Lamaze and parenting teacher, sometimes my students will call me at home if they are in labor and need a little help remembering how the breathing patterns go.

I was on the phone one afternoon helping a student breathe through a contraction when my pastor came unexpectedly to the front door. My then three-year-old son answered the door, and when my pastor asked where I was and what I was doing, my son calmly replied that "Mom was breathing heavy on the phone again. It's her job you know."

Thank goodness my pastor knew I was a Lamaze instructor!

Lynn Noelle Mossburg

8

ON MOTHERHOOD

I lost everything in the postnatal depression.

Erma Bombeck

My Previous Life

The greatest sight one sees beneath the stars is the sight of worthy motherhood.

George W. Truett

In my previous life, before I was reincarnated as a mother of three, I wore clothes that fit and matched. I wore makeup and curled my hair every day. I had my eyebrows waxed and my nails done. But no one gave me graham cracker kisses. No one ever told me how pretty I look in sweats.

In my previous life, I read *Time* magazine and the newspaper. My repartee of regular television viewing transcended *Arthur* and *The Magic School Bus,* and I devoured all the bestselling novels. But no one asked me to read *The Velveteen Rabbit* at bedtime. No one ever requested *The Little Engine that Could.*

In my previous life, I had a career and friends who were more than three feet tall. People asked for my opinions and entrusted me with important projects and confidential information. I had conversations where not once was mentioned snacks or potties or play dates. But no one asked me my favorite color or why the sky is so blue. No one ever wanted me to sing.

In my previous life, I *had* a life. I frequented aerobics classes, restaurants and the theater. I hosted parties where the themes had nothing to do with *Star Wars* or Winnie-the-Pooh. I shopped for myself and slept late on weekends. But no one made me Valentine cards. No one ever gave me dandelion bouquets.

In my previous life, I traveled, and my destinations did not hinge on theme parks or swimming pools or nap schedules. The Mayan ruins of the Yucatan, snorkeling in the Caribbean, museum hopping in Italy, Kabuki Theater in Japan . . . these were my playgrounds. I was the queen of the road and my destiny. But no one asked me to push the swing higher. No one ever invited me to splash in puddles or roll in the snow.

In my previous life, I held my emotions in check. I did not stomp my feet or grit my teeth. I could not easily be diminished to tears or tirades. I considered my demeanor as laid-back and easygoing. But, no one made me care enough to cry. No one ever just loved me, anyway.

In my previous life, I was free. I could carve my own path and follow my dreams. Nothing stood in my way. But the path was unsure and the vision blurred. No one ever gave me purpose enough to soar. Now, I endlessly rearrange piles of laundry, crumbs and toys. I am pulled and tugged, hassled and harassed, stepped on and sat upon, and desperate for some solitude. I am jean-clad and juice-stained, bleary-eyed and graying, underpaid and overwhelmed. And, sometimes I wonder who I am and what I've become. Then, one of my children shouts, "Mommy, I need you!" and it is perfectly clear.

I am the center of the Universe. I am MOM.

Gayle Sorensen Stringer

Good to Be Home

Years ago when my three boys were just wee ones, my old high-school friend, Marge, invited me to lunch at her home in a nearby upscale subdivision. She was a teacher, had never married and had recently purchased a condominium.

The minute I walked into her home, I knew there was something different about it, but I couldn't quite put my finger on what it was. I put my finger on the kitchen counter while admiring her tile, and realized what was so different. The counter wasn't sticky. Upon closer inspection, I saw that there wasn't any peanut butter oozing down the kitchen cabinets, no Kool-Aid puddle on the floor or cookie crumbs on the place mats. No one had left the half-gallon carton of milk out or put the mayonnaise back in the fridge without the lid.

After lunch, we sauntered into Marge's living room to sip our coffee and reminisce about the "good old days" and ponder "whatever happened to?" I was immediately struck by the fact that her stereo turntable cover didn't have fingerprints of assorted sizes all over it, and none of her records were warped from being used as Frisbees.

When Marge gave me directions to the bathroom, I made

my way up a flight of stairs which weren't covered with Hot Wheels tracks, slinky toys or yo-yos. Being the only female in a house with four males, I always approached bathrooms with caution. I carefully opened the door and there was no potty seat to be removed from the toilet. And—wonder of wonders!—the seat was down. I peeked behind the shower curtain, and there wasn't a turtle or frog to be seen in the tub—just a pretty bottle of perfumed bath crystals where usually I saw a soggy box of Soaky Fun Bubbles.

After a delightful afternoon of bringing each other up to date on our lives, I bade Marge good-bye, each of us promising the other that we would do this more often. I climbed into my clunky station wagon and headed home, wondering what series of crises would be reported to me by the sitter upon my arrival. It always seemed that when I treated myself to a day out, I was penalized by having to deal with all sorts of mishaps, spillage, clutter and fights that had occurred in my absence. The highway stretched before me, and I slowed my speed trying to put off the inevitable. I felt vaguely sorry for myself. I dawdled in the grocery store, not knowing what to get for dinner.

No one was in the yard when I pulled in, and the dogs didn't come out snapping at the grocery bag. It was suspiciously quiet inside the house, and I called out, "Where is everybody?"

"In the bathroom," came the reply.

"Great," I sighed. "What is it this time?"

When I went to the kitchen to deposit the groceries, it was noticeably free of dirty dishes and food morsels.

"We cleaned our room and the kitchen and now we're giving the dogs a bath," my eldest proudly proclaimed, as I approached the bathroom wondering what was going on.

Our two black Labrador retrievers were totally immersed in Soaky Fun Bubbles and, upon seeing me, leapt from the tub; two white clouds with white tails, knocked me to the sudsy floor, each bestowing a slurpy "welcome home" lick on my face. The three little boys and two big dogs thought this was wonderful entertainment, and we all slipped and slid around on the bathroom floor, bubbles everywhere, laughing hysterically.

I surveyed the ridiculous scene around me, and for some reason I couldn't explain, I felt sorry for Marge.

Jackie Fleming

THE FAMILY CIRCUS   By Bil Keane

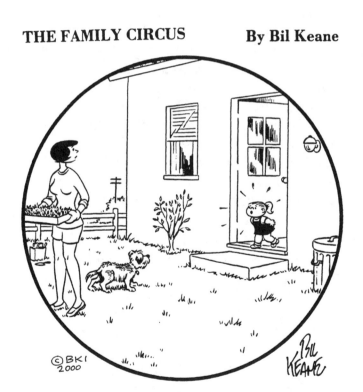

"The phone is ringing, the door bell is chiming, the dryer is busy and the oven is dinging."

Reprinted by permission of Bil Keane.

Everything Old Is New Again

The nicest thing about being a mother is that you get to relive your childhood. Everything becomes an adventure, whether it is chasing a cricket across the grass, going to the zoo or reading a favorite book, snuggled under the covers. Motherhood came easily to me, and I enjoyed the challenges of raising a family.

I am the mother of three boys: Phillip, my serious, intense six-year-old; Ryan, four, my little ray of sunshine; and my live-wire Adrien, who at eighteen months seems to have developed more ways of getting into trouble than a nine-arm octopus. They are the joy of my life and I have loved every roller-coaster day of being home with them. To our surprise and great joy, we recently found out that we are expecting another child. Since this is my fourth time around, I thought that I would not be fazed by an experience characterized by uncontrollable fatigue, hormone surges that would leave me in tears at the slightest upset, and bizarre urges to eat oranges at night, baked potatoes in the morning and curried chicken all day long. A miracle still, but an everyday miracle rather like the sun rising in the morning and setting at night.

Initially, we had thought to wait a few months before announcing it to our children, but Phillip, my little adult, sensed that something was provoking the whispered conversations with my mother and my girlfriends. Maybe he overheard me, maybe he read the title of my favorite dog-eared pregnancy handbook; either way, he turned to me one day and said: "I want a baby sister." And so the secret was out, and I couldn't have been happier about it.

However, I had hoped to postpone a serious discussion regarding the birds and the bees for a few more years, so I was unprepared to deal with the questions that my oldest two asked: "How did the baby get in your tummy, Mommy?" asked Ryan. Phillip, ever logical, wondered: "How is that baby going to come out?" I tried to give them the pat little answers that my mother had given me: a story about a little seed that the daddy plants, like a farmer plants a seed in the ground. Answers that Phillip did not want to accept. He wanted to know where Daddy got the seed and how he planted it, questions that delighted me with their inquisitiveness and stumped me because I did not know how much information was too much information. Finally, I decided to try and answer all questions as completely and truthfully as possible, and I found a book that contained diagrams of the male and female reproductive system, complete with pictures of the developing fetus.

This elicited a new round of questions and pretty soon became one of their favorite picture books. Phillip enjoyed the map-like diagrams and would trace the path the egg took in the fallopian tube and Ryan became absorbed in the babies' pictures, wondering if "our" baby looked like that. Upon learning, for instance, that a baby didn't start out with arms and feet but instead started out with a little tail, he became very alarmed at the thought that our baby might have one. He would ask me every day: "Mommy, does that baby still have a tail?" We would look at the development chart to see if it had grown legs yet. He wasn't reassured until my eight-week sonogram clearly showed little arm and leg buds. Now he wants to know if the baby is still growing, if I can feel it moving and could he feel it moving, too? He will sometimes rush up to me and for no reason kiss my protruding abdomen or put his hand on it to feel his baby kicking. Now that he has learned that the baby has ears, he sings to the baby. Phillip, on the other hand, is much more interested in the mechanics of birth and recently announced that he wanted to go to the hospital with me and watch the baby be born! I wish I could read Adrien's mind to see what is going on in his little head; undoubtedly, he must think that this is a lot of fuss over the fact that Mommy has much less lap room!

This pregnancy that was supposed to be so routine and ordinary appears fresh and new to me, like a lost toy suddenly found. I am experiencing impending motherhood through the eyes of my children, rediscovering things that I had forgotten, remembering the true miracle of birth, the wonder of feeling a child move within, the awe of a heartbeat, the sheer beauty of motherhood in full bloom. And my children are my teachers.

Francoise Inman

They'll Be Fine

I am a single mother of two. When my oldest child started school, I was like all mothers: I stood, at a loss for words, when he dashed to meet his new friends, without noticing that I was standing there waiting for my bye-bye hug. I felt as if someone just snatched him from me, and I would never have his full attention and dependence again.

I had a lot of time to share with my youngest child, who is three years younger than my oldest. I had him at my side tugging at my shirt strings for three years. Where I went, he went. He was by all means "my baby." We had a special bond, the two of us. He was my li'l man and I was so dependent on his being with me for such a long time that I dreaded the upcoming year for he would start school too. Every mother knows the hassles that come with shots for school, preschool records, little backpacks and the extra school supplies, not just for one but for two.

For a while, I was working the midnight shift. One day after seeing my oldest off to the bus, I came back into the house, and as the sitter left, Jeremy said to her, "Don't wowwy. I be good and go back to sweep wit Mommy." Back then, I would sleep for a few hours then get up and do the Mommy things. He would help me prepare supper since the earlier I cooked the more time I had with his brother. His brother would get off the bus, we would play for a while, then do homework, eat and bathe. By that time, it was almost time for bed and we would nestle up in our beds and retire for the evening. However I had to get up three hours later to get ready for work. By this time, the sitter would come. Jeremy heard her every time, and he would come into the living room where she would study before I went to work, and watch her or cartoons and then give the sweetest little kisses as I exited our home.

One morning I got home, changed out of uniform and slipped into the car. I figured I would try to get my errands done before retiring for a few hours sleep. I came home exhausted. I had run all over the malls for a certain crimson red T-shirt to match with Jeremy's little shorts that I had bought for him to wear to school. I searched and searched. My last stop was at Kmart. As I headed toward the children's department, up against the wall I noticed the perfect T-shirt. I grabbed it and started saying, "Look, Jeremy, look! Here is one and it's perfect." I turned around and he was gone. Knowing how children love to hide in between things, I started looking for him. I called out his name, but he never answered. Several minutes had passed, and I was panicking, screaming his name. An associate from the store approached me and asked me if I lost something. I screamed, "I can't find my baby! Someone has stolen my baby!!!" The manager summoned a clerk to call the police as they issued a code on a missing child. I rambled hysterically through the store looking for my baby.

By this time, a policeman was asking me questions. I was telling him that my son was standing beside me while I picked out his shirt. As I reached for a picture of him in my purse, the officer asked, "Ma'am, what was he wearing?"

I started telling him, little bitty white tennis shoes, blue jean shorts and a yellow T-shirt with . . . "Oh, my gosh!" I turned red with embarrassment.

The officer said, "Ma'am?"

I started to cry.

He asked, "Ma'am, what is it?"

I exclaimed, "I am so sorry!"

"What, Ma'am, what is it?"

I exclaimed, "He started kindergarten today!"

Honestly, I was so embarrassed that I paid for his shirt and went straight to the school and stood behind the glass of his new classroom. As I watched him playing with his new friends, I realized I was all by myself now, no one to call my name thirty times a day, ask questions of why and how come! I stood there remembering the time I first held him and his brother, and I started to cry.

The next day, I stood at their school doors and watched until the principal walked up to me, grabbed my hand and said, "Ma'am, I promise they will be fine!"

Patsy Hughes

Rhymes and Reasons

A household of children certainly makes other forms of success and achievement lose their importance by comparison.

Theodore Roosevelt

As I sang to my newborn son, I contemplated my decision. The tune soothed us both.

When I think about Patrick, my firstborn, I remember how difficult those first few months were. Whenever he got restless, I'd draw from my teaching days and sing a rhyme or two.

Patrick's first cry had been in late August—and so was the first day of school for my former students. I missed the cheerful faces of the schoolchildren and the musty smell of a classroom that had been closed up all summer. Had I made the right choice? Should I have continued teaching after having the baby? Would I lose contact with my teaching peers and fade into lost volumes of aging yearbooks?

As conflicted as I was, I knew seeing my young baby mature into a toddler and then a little boy was something

I did not want to miss. On snowy mornings past, I'd be scraping my windshield before work. Now I was cuddling my son under warm blankets and watching the snow fall. An afternoon at the museum, or a visit to the library story hour, or a walk around the block was very special for both of us. While most of my focus was on mother-child activities, I also found time to sew and read, luxuries that were virtually nonexistent before. I enjoyed making Patrick's pumpkin costume for Halloween and felt proud of his Christmas stocking, with the sequins I had worked so hard to apply, hanging on the fireplace mantel.

Unfortunately, we at-home moms are often misunderstood. I am asked, "Why are you wasting your life and career staying at home?" My reply is simple: "I can always go back to teaching, but never to those wonderful days of motherhood." What a sad commentary on society when the most important job in the world must be defended. It has been six years since I made this decision. It is just as special to see two more stockings above our fireplace (yes, with sequins, too!) and the costume gallery I have created since that first October.

I walked near my sons' room last night and listened to Anthony corral his imaginary puppies and Dominic wail for attention. I started to enter to comfort my little one, only to be pleasantly surprised by my oldest son singing those same rhymes from my teaching days to calm his littlest brother.

As I leaned against the door, a new song filled my heart. It was then I realized I hadn't given up teaching at all!

Antionette Ishmael

The Beholder's Eye

Shoving the vacuum into its home in the hall closet, I stifled a groan. A half-day of housework behind me and I still wasn't ready for the out-of-state company expected any minute. My four small children whirled through, leaving a wake of toys, crumbs and stray shoes scattered across the recently trackless carpet. And then I saw it: the sliding doors of the family room. The ones I had washed and scrubbed earlier that morning. Generous finger streaks and tiny nose prints mottled the freshly polished glass panes. *And that looks like . . .* Frowning, I stepped nearer and bent for a closer inspection. *Why, it is! Peanut butter and Oreo cookies smudged all over. Those kids!* Near tears, I plopped onto the couch and grabbed the jangling phone. "Hello?" I growled.

"Hello, dear," answered my mother from her own couch a state away. "Are you busy?"

"Oh, you have no idea!" I said, exasperated. "We're expecting guests and I just can't seem to get all the housework caught up around here and the kids . . ."

"That reminds me," she interrupted. "I should do some of my own. Housework, that is. The mirror above the couch is smeared. But, you know, every time I look at the sweet baby prints your little ones left there last month, I can't bring myself to wipe them away. After all, I'm still showing them off to my friends as 'priceless artwork!'" My gaze ping-ponged around the room. A half-eaten cracker here, wadded socks there, tilting towers of picture books in the corner. I grinned. Crowning it all was a hand-painted masterpiece on the patio doors. Unnumbered. One-of-a-kind. My own piece of priceless artwork.

Carol McAdoo Rehme

The Hug

The best thing to hold onto in life is each other.

Anonymous

It had been a long day already. And it was only three in the afternoon. My fourteen-month-old daughter, Lucy, was teething and we'd both been up all night—and all day. Nothing I did seemed to comfort her and I was getting more frustrated, closer to my wit's end. To top it off, my husband was out of town and the late August sun was making Lucy hot and sweaty, both of us more cranky. At the same time my heart ached for her, my head ached for aspirin.

By four o'clock, Lucy was whimpering about losing Barney under the couch and Elmo under the chair. Having rescued her stuffed animals, I hugged and rocked her. I carried her with one arm and went back to sponging mashed peas up off the tile kitchen floor, brown bananas from the crevices in her high chair. I thought about the graduate school classes I had left when she was born.

Before we had Lucy, I had sworn I'd never become one of those mothers who cleaned and cooked all day in their housecoats, their hair a mess, their feet in terrycloth slippers. But there I was, my hair looking like it had gone through the heavy heat cycle of the clothes dryer, my eyes bloodshot and puffy. I indeed was still in my bathrobe, and I hadn't showered.

Carrying Lucy, because she cried at my feet if I didn't, I sang to her as I cleaned up the kitchen, beginning with "Somewhere over the Rainbow" and resorting to "A Hundred Bottles of Beer on the Wall." Singing seemed to work. Lucy was calm until I got to bottle eighty-eight and then she let out a small whimper, which soon developed into tears. I gave up cleaning and patted her back. She was not to be consoled and let out a wail I was sure was going to alert the police.

I took Lucy for a walk, read her *Runaway Bunny* and tried tickling and playing our favorite games. Nothing was working. I tried singing again. Nothing. If ever I needed her to sleep, it was then. But every time I brought her near the crib in her room, she cried real tears, clutching at me, screaming "Nooooo."

As much as I longed to leave her there, as much as my body told me to do so, I couldn't. I stared at blue eyes rimmed with red as I brought her back into the kitchen and knew all she needed was rest. *Sleep, darn it,* a voice screamed in my head, something I would never reveal to my friends who have children.

By five o'clock, I stooped to Barney videos and chocolate ice cream. This brought me some reprieve. I collapsed on the couch beside her and wondered if I was doing something wrong, somehow falling short as a new mother.

Darkness came with me hardly noticing. I told myself that it was not a terrible thing to put my daughter to bed just a little early that night. We climbed the stairs together, Lucy and I, small petal fingers holding onto both of my hands high above her head. She let out a sigh at the top of the steps by her bedroom. "Me too, Lucy," I said softly, picking her up.

I lifted her onto the changing table, feeling more tired than I ever knew possible. I missed the wonderful glow, the bigger-than-life, stronger-than-any-words kind of love I felt for my daughter. I wasn't used to being so irritated and overwhelmed.

Both of us quiet, I put Lucy's Mickey Mouse pajamas on her. Silent and somewhat still, she stood on the changing table as I held her close to zip her up. I breathed in the clean smell of her hair, feeling blonde curls tickle my chin. A certain sadness tugged at me. This isn't what I thought motherhood to be.

Suddenly, Lucy reached her arms around my neck, holding the back of my head tight between her arms. Little hands, little everything, pulled me to her, and she pressed her cheek to mine. It took only a moment to realize what was happening. "She's hugging me, she's hugging me," I wanted to shout. "She's hugging me for the very first time." I wanted to yell for my husband, a neighbor, anyone to come see what my daughter was doing for the first time.

We held each other for a few seconds, my daughter standing on the changing table dressed in her fuzzy red sleeper, her arms around my neck, her cheek pressed to my left shoulder. "Oh, Lucy," I whispered, my words tight with tears. I never wanted to let go.

Lucy let go first and was onto her next discovery, ready to bed down with Piglet, Pooh and her favorite soft blanket. I stood next to the crib, looking down at her. She was so beautiful lying there, holding Pooh, blinking blue jewels at me. I stroked her forehead as I do each night and pulled the blanket up to her chin.

As I left her room, my time now all to myself, precious solitude didn't seem quite as important, the fatigue drifting from my shoulders. I was preoccupied with her very first hug and how lucky I was to have gotten it.

Martine Ehrenclou

Alone Time for Mom   ·

All I needed this morning was a half-hour alone, thirty minutes of peace and quiet to help preserve my sanity. No "Mom, do this," "Mom, I need that," "Mom, he hit me," "Mom, I spilled juice on the couch."

Just me, a hot Calgon bath, and nothingness.

I shouldn't dream so big. After getting the two oldest off to school, I settled the youngest in front of the television to watch *Barney and Friends* and said, "Honey, listen closely. Your mommy is going to crack. She's losing her marbles. She's teetering on the edge of permanent personality damage. This is because she has children. Are you following me so far?"

He nodded absently while singing, "Barney is a dinosaur from our imagination . . ."

"Good. Now, if you want to be a good little boy, you'll sit right here and watch Barney while Mommy takes a nice, hot, quiet, peaceful, take-me-away bath. I don't want you to bother me. I want you to leave me alone. For thirty minutes, I don't want to see you or hear you. Got it?"

Nod.

"Good morning boys and girls! . . ." I heard the purple wonder say.

I headed to the bathroom with my fingers crossed.

I watched the water fill the tub. I watched the mirror and window steam up. I watched the water turn blue from my bath beads. I got in.

I heard a knock on the door.

"Mom? Mom? Are you in there, Mom?"

I learned long ago that ignoring my children does not make them go away.

"Yes, I'm in here. What do you want?"

There was a long pause while the child tried to decide what he wanted.

"Um . . . can I have a snack?"

"You just had breakfast! Can't you wait a few minutes?"

"No, I'm dying! I need a snack right now!"

"Fine. You can have a box of raisins."

I heard him pad off to the kitchen, listened as he pushed chairs and stools around trying to reach the raisin shelf, felt the floor vibrate when he jumped off the counter, and heard him run back to the TV room.

"Hi, Susie! Can you tell me what color the grass is?" Barney asked from the other room.

Knock, knock, knock. "Mom? Mom? Are you in there, Mom?"

Sigh. "Yes, I'm still in here. What do you need now?"

Pause. "Um . . . I need to take a bath, too."

Right.

"Honey, can't you wait until I'm done?"

The door opened just a crack. "No, I really need to take one now. I'm dirty."

"You're always dirty! Since when do you care?"

The door opened all the way. "I really need to take a bath, Mom."

"No, you don't. Go away."

He stood in the middle of the bathroom and started taking off his pajamas.

"I'll just get in with you and take a bath, too."

"No! You will not get in with me and take a bath! I want to take my own bath! I want you to go away and leave me alone!" I began to sound like the three-year-old with whom I was arguing. He climbed onto the edge of the tub, balancing carefully, and said, "I'll just get in with you okay, Mom?"

I started to shriek, "No! That is not okay! I want my own bath, all by myself! I don't want to share! I want to be alone!"

He thought for a moment and said, "Okay. I'll just sit here and you can read me a book. I won't get in, Mom, until you're done." He flashed me a knockdown charming smile.

So I spent my morning-alone time reading *One Fish, Two Fish* to a naked three-year-old who sat on the edge of the tub with his chin resting on his knees, arms wrapped around his bent legs, slight smile on his face. Why fight it? It won't be long before I have all the alone time I want. And then I'll probably feel bad about not having any more together time.

Crystal Kirgiss

Let Me

God, please do not let me miss those moments that I could have spent with my child. Let me carry him more often and feel his tiny body gently wrapped in my loving arms. For someday I will not have the strength to pick him up anymore.

Let me hold him close to smell his freshly washed hair and breathe in that wonderful baby scent that covers his delicate skin, for surely he will not smell this deliciously sweet for very long.

Let me enjoy changing his diapers for this gives me the chance to play with his miniature toes, tickle his tummy and make him feel comfortable. Someday he will ask me to leave and shut the door behind me claiming he can manage by himself.

Let me take more walks with him in his stroller while I can look down at his little face that is staring in wonder at this new world all around him. Let me do this often, for soon he will be able to walk on his own and leave the safety of his carriage.

Let me stand beside his crib at night for longer than a moment to watch him surrender to his peaceful slumber.

These nights spent in a crib will be replaced soon enough by a much less cozy place for dreams.

Let me make him laugh every day. For I am sure the precious sounds of his first giggles are apt to change with time.

Let me delight in each and every milestone he reaches. Before I know it walking, drinking from a cup and other small miracles he has learned will seem ordinary.

Let me tell him how much I love him. Since there are bound to be times when he will not want to sit still to hear this.

Let me continue to listen attentively to him even after he has mastered the art of talking. Since people tend to listen less closely to a child once language becomes fluent.

Let me make time for peek-a-boo and pat-a-cake and other baby games. There will come a day when he will no longer want to participate in such childish antics.

Let me learn to enjoy the sound of him calling me "Mommy" even if it is yelled through the dripping of tears. For one day I will no longer be "Mommy" to him, but rather just "Mom."

Let me be the world to him right now because as every mother sadly comes to realize, their babies soon discover the world outside of their mother's arms.

Let me do these things and so much more, despite being busy, tired or overwhelmed because I would hate to look back and harbor regrets of times gone by that were lost to less important things than my son.

Yes, dear Lord, I want my son to grow up to be a strong, loving and intelligent man, but please Lord do not let this happen overnight because someday memories will be all I have.

Michelle Mariotti

Happy Birthing Day to Me

The birthday card is easy to find, but I see no anniversary card that's just right. I walk the rows in the card shop, fingering a card that waxes poetic on ten years of marriage, reading another that lauds twenty-five years of employment, and another that congratulates the founding of a business. Among the rows of sympathies, empathies, best wishes, get wells, birthdays and special occasions, I can not find a card honoring my imminent anniversary. Though my milestone is not acknowledged by retail symbols or spiritual rites, for me, the day marks a moment when I began my coming of age and my understanding of true unconditional love. This day, the birthday of my oldest daughter, is my anniversary of becoming a mother.

I was the first of my friends to get married and the first to get pregnant. The term "expanding horizons" took on new meaning: I watched with awe and alarm as my stomach ballooned. I felt a mixture of fascination and discomfort as my baby jostled and wrestled inside me. I watched other people's infants for clues: I swooned over babies peacefully teething in strollers, babies blissfully sleeping on their mom's shoulders, babies crowing over their food in restaurants. I imagined my child would have a

peaches-and-cream complexion and a personality as beautiful and compelling as a postcard of paradise. The sight of
my own feet became a distant dream and the image of my
newborn child and my own parenting prowess became a
constant vision.

Three days after my due date, I had a serious talk with
my unborn child. "We are ready for a closer relationship,"
I said, in what I hoped was a coaxing tone. "It's time to
come out."

I stretched the headphones over my stomach and
played a Sousa marching song instead of the usual
Mozart. I did an elephantine version of "thumping" jacks
and then trudged up and down the stairs enough times to
scale the Eiffel Tower. When I finally fell into bed, I felt like
a ship that could not find the right dock. I wiggled and
squirmed. I stole my sleeping husband's pillows so I could
cushion my belly. Just as I was getting drowsy, I felt mois-
ture spreading everywhere.

"Oh my, I'm leaking!" I shouted. The damp and the
noise rousted my husband. "Your waters have broken," he
said, quietly proud of his pre-parenting proficiency.

Suddenly, I was scared. What would it be like? Who
was this person I'd been growing for nine months?

Then a vice gripped my stomach and I stopped thinking. All to the way to the hospital and through the admis-
sion procedure, I tried to breathe between the pains. I
tried to imagine this child and our life together. But
mainly I bit my lip and tried not to make the paint peel off
the walls with my screaming.

The moment I saw my child, I forgot all pain. I was
seized with a wild, deep, fierce love. Every cell in me
reached out to this small splotched creature.

"Is that how she's supposed to look?" my husband
asked, as he cradled her. Her eyelids were streaked with
red, her skin yellowed, her hair dark and sparse.

"Yes," I said. "That is exactly how she's supposed to look."

In my vision of myself as a mom, I simply incorporate my child into my full and interesting life. The baby fits into my schedule as neatly as a long-lost puzzle piece.

This vision lasted for about three hours. I got her home from the hospital, fed her, struggled with getting the diaper to stay on, and held her until she fell asleep. Then I gingerly put her into her crib.

That's when it happened: "Did you see that?" I asked my husband. "She stretched!" I stood eagerly by, watching to see what else this miracle of a child could do. And in one way or the other, I have been standing by ever since.

Every year, I give my daughter a lovely birthday party. After one such glorious gathering, I sat in an exhausted heap among the puddles of ice cream and crumbs of cake. I sighed at the mounds of wrapping and ribbons. As I scooped a frosting flower off the cake plate, I suddenly realized that this day was not just my daughter's birthday: it was my anniversary of becoming a mother!

The anniversary of becoming a mother is one of the few life-changing moments that is rarely heralded. And whether our child is born to us or adopted, motherhood is a choice that permanently alters the way we view ourselves and our universe. It is the moment when we make a commitment to truly care for another human being. This vow goes beyond words or ceremony: this vow is etched in our cells and knitted into our hearts. I began looking for ways to acknowledge and celebrate this event and found none of the usual trappings: no designated card, no anniversary-of-a-mom flower bouquet or candy assortment. (Although, I imagine the card would have to be crayon smeared and hand-folded; the bouquet might be a motley array of daisies and dandelions, picked from other people's yards and the candy would feature pinched and half eaten chocolates, hastily shoved back into the box.)

Since there seemed few options for public ceremony (at the mere mention, my daughter looked at me with concern: I wasn't going to let this anniversary thing get in the way of her birthday, was I?), I began celebrating privately. I told my friends. I talked to my husband. I called my mom and recounted the story of my daughter's birth. The anniversary became a time of reflection and gratitude; a time to notice the richness of my role as a mother.

This year, I wake up with a sense of awe. "Happy anniversary," I say to myself as I look in the bathroom mirror. I imagine an auditorium filled with people. I hear the thunder of applause as I take the stage. The announcer's voice rings out, extolling, "Another year of service, another year of rigorous training, another year of trying hard, another year of flexibility (at this moment the announcer checks her notes.). "Actually," she says, "only five months of being really flexible." The crowd cheers and I see my daughter, waving and whistling from the audience. She is a course of study from which I never want to graduate; she is my deepest lesson in the art of love. I look into her eyes as I tell the crowd, "And here's to many, many more years."

Deborah Shouse

Seems Like Yesterday

Seems like yesterday . . .
The pains started.
I grabbed my bulging belly
And danced with your Papa
Shouting "It's time! It's time!"

Seems like yesterday . . .
You made your debut
Red-faced and screeching.
Your cries changed to coos as I held you.
My tears changed to oohs as you held me
Spellbound with your magical, wiggly humanness.
Yesterday we were one.
Today we were two.

Seems like yesterday . . .
Your middle-of-the-night colicky cries.
We went on our familiar walk
Down the stairs,
Through the living room,
The dining room,
The kitchen,

Into the pantry,
With made-up songs
Of soups and stews, pots and pans,
And back again.
Over and over.
Ten, twenty, a hundred times,
Until your cries were silenced.
Your breathing calmed.

Seems like yesterday . . .
Your first splashy sink bath.
Your first mushy meal.
Your first wobbly walk.
Your first wide-eyed word—
"Mama."

Seems like yesterday . . .
Your first birthday
Dressed in a diaper and frosting.
I helped you tear off wrapping paper,
Made your new teddy dance.
You threw down teddy
And had a party with the paper.

Seems like yesterday . . .
You were a bumblebee
At the dance recital.
The other bees buzzed
And floated and flitted onstage.
You stood frozen
Staring at the audience
Not moving a muscle
'Til the bow.
Then how you bowed and bowed and bowed.
And I clapped and clapped and clapped
'Til a man three rows back asked me to stop.

Seems like yesterday . . .
Your first day of school.
We played jumprope in the driveway
'Til the school bus came
And swallowed you up.
I wore the jumprope as a necklace
All morning long,
Through my chores,
Through my tears,
'Til you returned with kisses,
Smiles, and stories
Of what a grand place
Kindergarten was.

Seems like yesterday . . .
You wiggled out your first tooth.
Got your first hit in T-ball.
Slept overnight at a friend's
For the very first time.

Seems like yesterday . . .
You won the spelling bee.
The school's.
The county's.
The state's.
We flew to Washington, D.C.
So giddy and giggly we didn't need a plane.
We filled four days with memorials, monuments,
Memories for a lifetime.
It didn't matter that you misspelled "merganser"
In the first round.

Seems like yesterday . . .
You had your first date
And your first pimple
All on the same day.
I sat on the floor
Outside the locked bathroom door
'Til your tears stopped
And you let me make everything okay
Like Mamas are supposed to.

Seems like yesterday . . .
You got your driver's license.
Had your first fender-bender.
Went to your first prom.

Seems like yesterday . . .
When my own Mama died.
Everyone was kind,
Tried to say the right things.
Only you knew what to do.
You grabbed an armful
Of your Grammy's clothes—her nightgown, bathrobe,
     a dress.
We wrapped ourselves in her scent
And pored over old photos
Crying and laughing 'til dawn.

Seems like yesterday . . .
We drove you to college
Two states away.
The next day you called—collect,
And said you'd cried
For three hours after we'd left.
I understood. I cried for six.

Seems like yesterday . . .
You were my baby.
Now you're having your own baby.
Still, you will always be my baby.
Always.
Even when your baby's baby has a baby.
You will always be my baby,
And it will always seem like yesterday.

Lynn Plourde

A Perfect Gift for a
Not So Perfect Mother

Don't expect the best gifts to come wrapped in pretty paper.

H. Jackson Brown

Mother's Day, 5:00 A.M. From the fog of my dreams I hear the annoying buzz of the alarm clock. I feel a flash of sympathy for my husband at having to get up at such an early hour. But slowly the fog clears, and I realize that the alarm is for me. I edge one leg toward the side of the bed but the chilly morning air sends me back to the warm softness of my covers. The snooze alarm is working overtime, and my husband gives me a subtle push. Finally I'm in motion.

While most other mothers are still asleep, dreaming of breakfast in bed and flowers, I'm racing the clock to get ready for work. This Sunday is like any other Sunday at the hospital where I work the day shift; no time off for good behavior. No special recognition for all the nights I've gotten up with sick children, the hours I spent helping with homework (and I thought I was done with homework when I graduated from college), and all the meals I fixed that were greeted with "We have to eat this?" In the kitchen I gulp my coffee and contemplate my motherhood report card. For raising my lively thirteen-year-old, I've definitely earned a B+. She is thoughtful, kind and still has a sense of humor despite entering the rocky waters of adolescence. As for my younger daughter, I surely deserve an A for effort. But for results, I probably needed to repeat the course. This was my child who regularly offered to send her food to the hungry kids in China because my cooking was "too gross" for her to eat. When I picked her up after school, she frequently greeted me with a look that clearly said, "Oh, you're still my mother. I thought surely someone would realize that a mistake had been made and replace you." Oh, but I was good for something. Whenever I wore a piece of clothing or jewelry that she liked, she would declare, "I'll have that."

My thoughts were interrupted by footsteps on the stairs. Not the heavy tread of my husband, or the two-steps-at-a-time pace of my thirteen-year-old. This was the half-awake shuffle of my youngest, unaccustomed to being up at such an early hour. She moved down the steps, wearing a T-shirt that said "I Don't Do Mornings." How fitting.

She crawled into my lap, her long, lean legs hanging awkwardly over the edge of the chair. I tucked her silky head under my chin. The girls were getting so big and it seemed like so long since I'd held them. I had forgotten how good they smelled when they first woke up. After a few minutes she announced the reason for her early morning visit. "I've come to tell you Happy Mother's Day and I love you. I didn't have any money to buy you a present."

Flowers would only wilt, and breakfast in bed just led to the lingering smell of burnt toast in the house and crumbs in the sheets. But her early morning visit was a gift I would always treasure, and it reaffirmed my faith in my abilities as a mother. Perhaps I had passed the motherhood test after all!

I helped my little one back upstairs and tucked her back into bed. The soft smile on her lips quickly faded as her breathing became slow and deep. I tiptoed out the front door, a smile on my face and her gift in my heart.

Kyle Louise Jossi

That Day

"What was the best day of your life, and what was the worst?" I remember playing that game with some friends on the way to a ladies conference a couple of years ago. Memories ran long as every detail was recounted. Laughing to the point of tears, the minutes raced by as we relived our labor and delivery stories.

"What was the worst day of your life?" I pondered that question for a long time. My life had been fairly steady up until that point, no lows ever outweighing the highs. I wouldn't have trouble if I were asked that same question today. Just six months after that trip, I was shaken to my very core.

It was a cool spring day, and along with that little nip in the air were balloons, streamers and the giggly voices of fifteen precious children. The whole Mainse family was together for a birthday party for Rebekah, the youngest of the grandchildren, who was just turning a year old. This was not going to be a pool party, as was the custom, for the crispness in the air demanded jackets not bathing suits. Besides that, the pool, which had just been filled the week before, was a chilly sixty-five degrees and the gate was in the mandatory closed position. But that didn't seem to dampen the mood as the swing-set was full and balls and balloons were flying everywhere.

The party hadn't officially started yet but the children were quite happy just being together. The adults were, too, as they sipped coffee in the family room, mindful of the youngest children playing in the basement.

Sitting on a couch together, my husband Ron and I were deep into conversation. I asked him if he wanted a cup of coffee. This was unusual because he was not a big coffee drinker; one cup in the morning was more than enough. Yet, almost without hesitation, he said yes.

As I walked to the kitchen, I heard the laughing and squealing from outside growing louder. I smiled as I gazed out the window at the happy faces. As I took a mug out of the cupboard, my gaze fell again on the backyard. This time it stopped on the gate to the pool area—the open gate. Quickly, I scanned the pool and deck around it and saw no one. Relieved, I called to my husband to go out and close the gate. Even though the solar blanket was covering the water, the thought of children playing a few feet away was unsettling to me.

Reluctantly, Ron got up, tearing himself away from the conversation. I watched from the kitchen window as he sauntered outside, petting the dogs and tickling the children as he went. Finally, he reached the gate. As I poured the coffee, he pulled the gate toward him. He stopped. And so did I. Slowly, almost hesitantly, I watched Ron walk over to the edge of the pool. Puzzled, I stood, still holding the coffee cup in my hands.

The next few seconds felt like they were in slow motion. I watched from the kitchen window as Ron slowly pulled back the solar blanket. Suddenly, fully clothed, he jumped into the pool. My whole body went numb as I watched in horror as he lifted the limp body of our two-and-a-half-year-old son from the water.

Now I was on fast forward. I screamed like I had never screamed before, dropped the mug of coffee, and yelled,

"Eric's in the pool!" My legs had a mind of their own. I had to be out there. I ran through the kitchen to the nearest door and fought with it for what seemed like forever until I realized it was locked. Finally, I flung it open as hard as my strength would allow and ran across the yard. I was vaguely aware of adults screaming and running behind me.

By the time I reached the pool, Ron and Eric were at the edge of the shallow end. Eric was ashen white with bloody water coming from his mouth and nose. But that's not all that was coming from his mouth. Crying. Beautiful crying. With that sound it felt like all of the energy drained from me and I slumped against the fence, sobbing uncontrollably. He was alive.

After Eric had thrown up an incredible amount of water, we stripped him, wrapped him in blankets, and took him to the emergency room. They took him right away, ran a number of tests, and kept him for a few hours for observation.

Today, Eric is a healthy, active four-year-old. Amazingly enough, one of his favorite pastimes is jumping off the diving board and swimming in the pool.

Thinking back, I can't help wondering "what if?" What if I hadn't suggested coffee to Ron? What if he hadn't accepted? What if I didn't notice the open gate? What if Ron didn't notice what looked to be a bird or raccoon under the pool blanket and hadn't gone over to investigate?

That day, one year ago, God not only saved our little boy's life, but he did something just as important. He left his mark on it. Almighty God obviously and deliberately intervened in the life of our little family, leaving no doubt that he is in control.

Yes, today playing that game would be easy. You see, in a few short minutes, the worst day of my life also became the best.

Ann Mainse

I Wonder Now, What Moment

I wonder now, what moment, what year it was, what
    day . . .
When the word he called me, "Mommy," just simply
    went away?
He was my little boy then, when that title was once
    mine . . .
When his smile was so contagious. When his sweet blue
    eyes would shine.

When he started kindergarten, it seems like yesterday . . .
"Please don't leave me, Mommy," I heard my little boy
    say.
"I love you, Josh. Don't worry. It's gonna be okay,"
As I headed to the classroom door and slowly walked
    away.

The tears streamed down my face as I stumbled down
    the hall,
"Mommy?" I heard him ask for me. "Mommy!" I heard
    him call.
And at that moment in my life, the word became so
    bittersweet . . .
I still see his face, so angelic, his hair as blonde as wheat.

As he got a little older and in his room at play,
With his little brother at his side, I overheard him say,
"Our Mommy is a writer. She'll be famous some day."
I smiled to realize, through his eyes, the picture I'd
    portray.

The things little boys are prone to do he also did for me,
The weeds he picked as flowers . . . his face was etched
    with glee.
With dirt-streaked cheeks and beaming eyes, he was a
    sight to see,
More precious than red roses were those weeds he
    picked for me.

And time again betrayed me as it stole the years away,
He'd speak, yet rarely did I hear the words he had to
    say.
He must have called me "Mommy" then, a thousand
    times or more,
But I really wasn't listening as I headed out the door.

Deadlines beckoned to me, and the rat race seemed
    appealing,
And blinded by my story lines I never saw time stealing,
Those priceless moments when little boys are small
    enough to play.
Oh, only if I could go back to taste one yesterday.

One day I overheard him say to someone on the phone,
"My mother is a writer now. She leaves me here alone.
But that's okay. I'm on my way. I'll soon be on my own."
And suddenly my eyes could see a boy who's almost
    grown.

Dear God, please? Could I go back? To hear the things
    he'd say?

To share his dreams? To kiss his cheek? To wipe his tears
away?
To touch his face? To hold his hand? Dear God, could I
erase,
Those years I wasted needlessly and put time back in
place?

As he graduates from high school, it seems like
yesterday . . .
When he was a little boy consumed with carefree play.
"I love you, Mom. Don't worry. It's gonna be okay.
He said before he headed for life's door and walked
away.

And still I weep for all those years floating on the winds
of time,
For all the days and moments when a little boy was
mine.
Yet my longing is so futile, for in that little boy's place,
A young man stands to kiss away the tears upon my
face.

I wonder now, what moment, what year it was, what
day . . .
When the word he called me, "Mommy," just simply
went away?
He was my little boy then, when that title was once
mine . . .
When his smile was so contagious. When his sweet blue
eyes would shine.

Lori Elmore-Moon

$\overline{9}$

EXPECTANT WISDOM

*B*efore becoming a mother I had a hundred theories on how to bring up children. Now I have seven children and one theory: Love them, especially when they least deserve to be loved.

Kate Samperi

If I Were Starting My Family Again

The words burst from the man sitting across from me, his eyes pleading for help. "What should I have done differently? If your children were young again, what would you do?" He was suffering the empty, deathlike feeling of a man whose children have strayed. He felt he had failed as a father.

His questions stayed with me. What insights had I gleaned from my own experience as a parent and from my years of counseling others? If I were starting my family again, what would I do to improve relations with my children? After some reflection, I jotted down the things I considered most important.

I would love my wife more. In the closeness of family life it is easy to take each other for granted and let a dullness creep in that can dampen the deepest love. So I would love the mother of my children more—and be more free in letting them see that love. I would be more faithful in showing little kindnesses—placing her chair at the table, giving her gifts on special occasions, writing her letters when I'm away. I have found that a child who knows his parents love each other needs little explanation about the character of God's love or the beauty of sex. The love between father and mother flows visibly to him and prepares him to recognize real love in all future relationships. When a mother and father join hands as they walk, the child also joins hands. When they walk separately, the child is slow to join hands with anyone. Sentimentalism? Then we need a lot more of it. Often there is too much sentiment before marriage and too little afterward.

I would develop feelings of belonging. If a child does not feel that he belongs in the family, he will soon find his primary group elsewhere. Many who live in the same household are worlds apart. Many children see their father only at the dinner table. Some never see him for days at a time. For others, father-child time together may be only a few minutes a week.

I would use mealtimes more to share the happenings of the day, instead of hurrying through them. I'd find more time for games or projects in which all could join. I would invite my children to become involved in the responsibilities and work of the family. When a child feels he belongs to the family, he has a stability, which can stand against the taunts of the gang and the cries of the crowd.

I would laugh more with my children. It has been said that the best way to make children good is to make them happy. I see now that I was, many times, too serious. While my children loved to laugh, I, too often, must have conveyed the idea that being a parent was a perennial problem. I remember the humorous plays our children put on for us, the funny stories they shared from school and the times I fell for their tricks and catch questions. Such happy experiences enlarged our love, opened the door for doing things together—and still bind us together. I would be a better listener. To most of us, a child's talk seems like unimportant chatter. Yet, I now believe, there is a vital link between listening to the child's concerns when he is young and the extent to which he will share his concerns with his parents when he is in his teens.

If my children were small again, I'd be less impatient if they interrupted my newspaper reading. There's a story about a small boy who tried repeatedly to show his father a scratch on his finger. Finally his father stopped reading and impatiently said, "Well, I can't do anything about it, can I?" "Yes, Daddy," the boy said. "You could have said, 'Oh.'"

I was once with a father who did not answer when his young son called to him again and again. "It's only the kid calling," the man said. And I thought it would not be long until the father will call the son and he will say, "It's only the old man calling."

I would give more encouragement. Probably nothing stimulates a child to love life and seek accomplishment more than sincere praise when he has done well.

I know now that encouragement is a much better element of discipline than blame or reprimand. Fault-finding and criticism rob a child of self-reliance, while encouragement builds self-confidence and moves a child on to maturity. Deep in human nature is the craving to be appreciated. And when those we love meet this need we will also grow in other graces.

So if I were starting my family again, I would persist in daily praise, seeing not only what the child is now, but also what he can be. I would seek to share God more intimately. We are not whole persons when we stress only the physical, social and intellectual. We are spiritual beings. And if the world is to know God and his will, parents must be the primary conveyors. For my part, I would strive to share my faith with my children, using informal settings and unplanned happenings. Rather than discuss abstract theology or impose rigid rules of family worship, I would pay more attention to the things my child notices and to what concerns him and find in these a natural way to discuss spiritual truths.

There is a story of a schoolmaster who once was asked: "Where, in your curriculum, do you teach religion?" "We teach it all day long," he replied. "We teach it in arithmetic by accuracy; in language by learning to say what we mean; in history by humanity; in geography by breadth of mind; in astronomy by reverence; in the playground by fair play. We teach it by kindness to animals, by good manners to one another and by truthfulness in all things."

I remember a little fellow, frightened by lightning and thunder, who called out one dark night, "Daddy, come. I'm scared." "Son," the father said, "God loves you and he'll take care of you." "I know God loves me," the boy replied. "But right now I want somebody who has skin on." If I were starting my family again, that is what I would want to be above all else—God's love with skin on.

John Drescher

Children Are . . .

Amazing, acknowledge them.
Believable, trust them.
Childlike, allow them.
Divine, honor them.
Energetic, nourish them.
Fallible, embrace them.
Gifts, treasure them.
Here now, be with them.
Innocent, delight with them.
Joyful, appreciate them.
Kindhearted, learn from them.
Lovable, cherish them.
Magical, fly with them.
Noble, esteem them.
Open-minded, respect them.
Precious, value them.
Questioners, encourage them.
Resourceful, support them.
Spontaneous, enjoy them.
Talented, believe in them.
Unique, affirm them.
Vulnerable, protect them.

Whole, recognize them.
Xtraspecial, celebrate them.
Yearning, notice them.
Zany, laugh with them.

Meiji Stewart

THE FAMILY CIRCUS   **By Bil Keane**

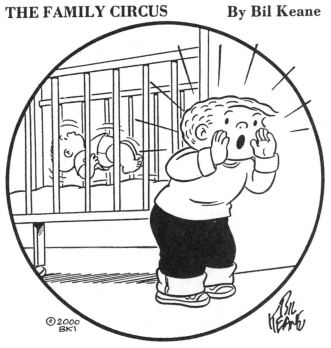

"Yeah, he's still sleeping."

Fantasy and Reality Clash with Birth of New Baby

Fantasies play an important role in our lives, fueling hope and helping us believe in the possibilities of the future. While pregnant with my first child, I attended a series of lectures at Piedmont Hospital. At one of them a pediatrician spoke and showed us slides. "Now I'm sure you all have contemplated your life with a baby," he said. "You dream of resting under the oak tree in the front yard, the beautiful baby sleeping peacefully by your side while you sip a cold glass of lemonade. Here is the reality."

He flashed a slide of a screaming, red-faced, runny-nosed infant with its tiny fists balled up in our personal fantasies. *Not my baby*, we thought.

Reality quickly sets in when we become parents. But we don't lose our capacity to fantasize. It's just that our initial fantasies change and we develop new ones. Here are some examples of my own.

Maternity Leave

Fantasy: Maternity leave will be a period lasting several months, consisting of blissful bonding with the new baby, and in my spare time, sewing balloon shades for the nursery, sending out engraved birth announcements with long letters to all the out-of-town friends and finally organizing photos from the past two years.

Reality: I have no choice but to bond with my daughter because she nurses for forty-five minutes every two hours. However, blissful is not the word to describe sitting on my couch for ten hours a day with my blouse hanging open. There is little time left for anything else besides laundry and changing diapers. The birth announcements are fill-in-the-blank ones my husband buys at the drugstore, and I find myself wishing I'd given my daughter a name shorter than Catherine Hamilton.

New fantasy: Getting to take a shower and eat lunch in the same day, and possibly getting out of my nightgown before noon.

Marriage After Children

Fantasy: Tom and I will become a joyful unit, more in love than ever as we sit peacefully at the dinner table, contemplating the beautiful baby we have created, and spending many happy hours dreaming of our future as a family.

Reality: My daughter thinks the initial clink of silverware on my plate is her signal it's time to nurse.

New fantasy: My fantasy involves men developing the ability to breast-feed. I'm not sure what my husband's fantasy is, but I notice that he spends a lot of time looking at the Victoria's Secret Catalog, where the women don't have stretch marks and I'm sure never suffered mood swings caused by postpartum hormonal imbalances.

Mothering

Fantasy: Although I know it will be difficult, I will maintain my composure at all times and will never yell at my children, an act that can damage their delicate psyches.

Reality: In addition to their ability to be incredibly cute and adorable, children have the capacity to make even the most patient person crazy at times when they do things like hide the car keys in the dishwasher or throw your watch down the toilet.

New fantasy: That the doors and windows will be closed and the neighbors away when I discover things my children have done, such as dumping a five-pound sack of flour on the floor and trying to clean it up by spraying it with Lysol. The result is that my kitchen floor looks like a relief map of the Rocky Mountains and smells like the bathroom at the bus station.

Food for the Family

Fantasy: I will have plenty of time to focus on the nutritional needs of my family and I will prepare complete, balanced meals every night the way my mother did.

Reality: There are days when finding the time to heat up a hot dog is a challenge.

New fantasy: That McDonald's will add carrot sticks to Happy Meals so I can pretend that they are nutritionally balanced.

I believe in the power of fantasy. It allows me to face the future, knowing that in less than four years I will have a teenager in the house. But I'm not worried. I know my daughter will continue to be polite, maintain open communication with me and will never be embarrassed by anything I say or do. Yeah right!

Jan Butsch

United States of Motherhood

The luminous numbers clicked as the time moved from 1:59 A.M. to 2:00 A.M. I shifted the weight on my lap and moved my son from one breast to the other.

Michael quickly made it clear that he was no longer interested in nursing. I moved him to my shoulder and patted his warm little back, waiting for that satisfying burp that would signal his stomach's acceptance of my late-night offering. Beneath me, I felt my legs growing numb and tingly. Even with a cushion, this wooden rocker was painful to sit in for long periods, night after night.

From the light of the streetlamp, I could see shadows in my son's room. The quiet of the evening settled around us, but still Michael wouldn't sleep. "Colic," said the pediatrician. "We don't know why it happens. He'll grow out of it in about three months. We suspect their digestive systems start to mature by then. You're home free the day he passes gas. Sorry."

Sorry? Sorry? My patience and my body were worn thin. All the baby books had profiled an infant who would spend most of his early first year snoozing.

With my Southern Hemisphere sporting more stitches

than a Quaker's sampler and my hair coming out in chunks, I was a poster child for postpartum distress. My sanity began to unravel as I hallucinated that I was part of an ancient Mayan culture where babies were gourds. The next day, when I dragged myself, baby and car seat in tow, into the pediatrician's office, I had been up forty-eight hours straight. Michael had slept a mere forty-five minutes during that two-day eternity. Thirty of those forty-five minutes had been on the car ride to the clinic. If I could only stay awake long enough, I might be able to drive to Alaska and back in three months.

The drugs to ease Michael's system began, thank goodness, to take effect. His naps fell into a general pattern, though their duration was far shorter than the experts led me to believe. But nighttime was party time for Mr. Mike. I read books that extolled the virtues of letting him scream. I listened to tapes by experts telling me to walk away. I tried gizmos and gadgets that shook his bed and me like a blender on high speed. But I couldn't walk away or relegate him to machinery. He was obviously in distress. The least I could do, I reasoned, was sit with him through the long and painful nights while he squirmed and struggled to fall asleep.

So we rocked. We rocked the circumference of the Earth. Then we rocked our way to the moon. Tonight we had been rocking toward Pluto. I brushed the velvety crown of his head. So dear, so soft, like chick down. I curled and uncurled his tiny fingers. I struggled with my anger. I sat there alone with him as my husband slept. Why wasn't the baby sleeping? How long could I go without rest? A wave of shame broke over me. Wasn't I blessed to have him? Wouldn't a million women give anything to be holding a child? Then, as I glimpsed the moon moving behind a cloud, a thought came to me. A million women. A million mothers. A million babies.

Suddenly I realized that I was not alone. All over the globe, women were holding their babies. Some were lucky enough to sit in rockers. Some crouched on the ground. Some had a roof over their heads, as I did. Many more were exposed to the elements, shielding their babies from the rain, the snow, the sun.

We were all alike. We held our children and prayed. Some would not live to see their children grown. Some children would not live out the year. Some would die of hunger. Some from bullets or sickness.

But for a moment, under the same pale moon, we were all together. Rocking our babies and praying. Loving them and hoping.

From that night on, I viewed my time with Michael differently. The fatigue never left me. The seat never seemed any softer. But as I sat with him, I felt the company of a million women, a billion women—mothers, all, holding our babies in our arms.

Joanna Slan

Surviving the Early Years of Momhood

As a woman you will never experience anything as wonderful as motherhood. There will be many hurdles along the way, such as colic, breast-feeding, eating solid food, temper tantrums and the first day of school. These are all challenging both for baby and mother. I will start with my least favorite.

The Colic Hour

Colic, as described by doctors, is a spasm of the intestines that causes pain. I can tell you from firsthand experience, colic is torture, for both the baby and mother. Colic most often presents itself at the same time each day. In my son's case, it was at dinnertime. I spent many nights walking my son around the room while trying to snatch bites of my cold dinner. (Notice I said walking around the room.) I'm not sure why babies prefer walking, but they do. Their little brains seem to know as soon as you sit down. You can try to trick them by continuing the bouncing motion produced by walking, but it rarely works. It is as if the baby can sense it and says, "I told you to walk me around the room, and I meant it." You will comply, and he knows it. At this point, you are beginning to be wrapped around your child's little finger.

On Breast-Feeding

Breast-feeding is a joyous experience. In this case, reading helpful books is acceptable and recommended. What you want to steer clear of is advice-giving friends and family. They will bombard you with comments such as, "How do you know if he's getting enough?" Or, "I think he is eating too much. He will get fat." Or the famous, "Why don't you try a pacifier instead?" Turn a deaf ear to these comments. You and your baby will know what to do. Submerge yourself in the feeling. Look into his eyes. Talk to him. Savor every minute. (The colic hour is quickly approaching.)

Milestones—To Read or Not to Read

Soon, your baby will encounter many milestones. During this period, reading can be good or bad. Avoid the articles that describe what your baby should be doing at a certain age. These are only good if he is really doing the activities they describe. If he is not, you will start saying, "My baby is not doing those things yet, maybe there is something wrong." Ignore what the books are saying. You don't need the concern.

Do They Really Need Solid Food?

When your baby starts eating you will need a large bib, lots of paper towels, and a floor mat for the over-zealous eater. He will soon become bored with strained foods. It is time to introduce the chunky variety. Along with this comes the dreaded fear of choking. Try to avoid mashing your baby's food. Your baby needs to learn how to chew. For my son's first few feedings I'll admit, I stood by ready to deliver the Heimlich maneuver at the first sign of trouble. Remember, babies have fantastic gag reflexes and use them proficiently to avoid this mishap. I discovered this as I was pulling my son from his high chair, ready to deliver a firm back blow. In the time it had taken me to free him from his confines, he had dislodged the offender. So sit back and enjoy the show.

Baby's First Words

If you find that your child's first word is "NO" instead of "Mommy" or "Daddy," do not be alarmed. Your child learns from imitating. As he begins to toddle, you will find yourself repeating the word "no" frequently. "No, don't touch." "No, it's hot." "No, it's sharp." You get the idea. To counteract this, repeat the words "I love you" to him often. I used the phrase, "Mommy loves you." Consequently, my son's first sentence was, "Mommy loves you."

The Temper Tantrum

Temper tantrums are a test of wills! Read all you can on this subject from the experts. In my experience, ignoring the tantrum was the best solution. Now, that is not always easy when you are in a crowded grocery store. At all costs do not give in. Your child is very smart. He will quickly learn what decibel range of a red-faced scream it will take for Mom to give in. If ignored long enough, the child will discover tantrums do not get him what he wants. So, if tantrums happen to you, tune them out. This, too, shall pass.

The Independent Child

By age three and four, you will notice a welcome change. Your child can now express his likes and dislikes very well. You can reason with a child of this age and teach him acceptable behavior. However, if you see him struggling with a project, try to avoid doing it for him. He will usually snap, "I can do it myself." As a mother, this will hurt your feelings. Try to remember this is a good thing. You will be grateful in the years to come when he becomes a self-sufficient youngster. At the same time he is testing his independence, he is also struggling with it. Hugging and cuddles are at an all-time high now. Eat it up! Savor every hug. There are few things more precious.

Kindergarten! Is It Really Necessary?

Hopefully, by age five you have weathered many storms and come out relatively unscathed. Starting kindergarten is more traumatic for the mother than it is for the child. I will admit I became slightly neurotic at this stage. (My family and friends would say very neurotic.) The thought of my son going off to school for the whole day made my blood run cold. How could I survive all day without him? Well, survive it I did, but not without a lot of tears. It is very important not to show your desire to throw yourself in front of the bus as it pulls away with your child inside. A more appropriate thing to do is to hop in the car and follow it! (Just to make sure he gets there all right.) Don't tell your husband if you do, however. He is sure to think you have gone off the deep end. If you need to tell someone, tell your mom; she will understand.

This is as far as I can go with my story. The future remains a mystery to me. I look forward to each new challenge with anticipation. There is only one thing I am sure of—I will love my son through good times and bad, more than I have ever loved anyone.

Jacqueline D. Carrico

Who Are Harder to Raise . . . Boys or Girls?

If you want to stir up a hornet's nest, just ask mothers, "Who are harder to raise—boys or girls?"

The answer will depend on whether they're raising boys or girls.

I've had both, so I'll settle the argument once and for all. It's girls.

With boys you always know where you stand. Right in the path of a hurricane. It's all there. The fruit flies hovering over their waste can, the hamster trying to escape to cleaner air, the bedrooms decorated in Early Bus Station Restroom.

With girls, everything looks great on the surface. But beware of drawers that won't open. They contain a three-month supply of dirty underwear, unwashed hose and rubber bands with blobs of hair in them.

You have to wonder about a girl's bedroom when you go in to make her bed and her dolls have a look of fear and disbelief in their eyes.

A mother once wrote me to agree. She said that, "after giving birth to three boys, I finally got a girl on my fourth try. At first, she did all the sweet little things I longed to see. She played coy, put her hands to her face when she laughed and batted her eyes like Miss Congeniality. Then she turned fourteen months and she struck like a hurricane. When she discovered she could no longer sail down the banister and make my hair stand on end, she turned to streaking. I'd dress her ever so sweetly and go to the breakfast dishes. Before one glass was washed, she'd strip, unlock the door and start cruising the neighborhood. One day, the dry cleaner made a delivery and said, 'my goodness, I hardly recognized Stacy with her clothes on.'

As she got older, she opened her brother's head with a bottle opener for taking her dolls and called the school principal a 'thug' to his face.

I am pregnant again. I sleep with a football under my pillow each night."

I knew of another mother, who said, "Boys are honest. Whenever you yell upstairs, 'What's all that thumping about?' you get an up-front reply, 'Joey threw the cat down the clothes chute. It was cool.'

When my daughter is upstairs playing with her dolls I yell, 'What are you girls doing?' She answers sweetly, 'Nothing.'

I have to find out for myself that they're making cookies out of my new bath powder and a $12.50 jar of moisturizer.

Her pediatrician advised me to 'not notice' when she insisted on wearing her favorite outfit for four months. How do you ignore a long dress with a ripped ruffle, holes in the elbow and a Burger King crown? How would you handle it if you were in a supermarket and the loudspeaker announced, 'Attention Shoppers. We have a small child in produce wearing a long pink dress with a gauze apron, glittery shoes and a Burger King crown.'? Our third child was born recently. Another girl. I told the orderly to pass maternity and go straight to geriatrics. I rest my case. God knows it's the only rest I've had in six years."

Whether mothers want to believe it or not, they compete with their daughters. They recognize in them every feminine wile in the book because they've used it themselves. It worked on "Daddy" when you used it, and it'll work again with your daughter. ("Daddy, you do believe that a tree can swerve right out in front of a car, don't you?")

Girls mature faster than boys, cost more to raise, and statistics show that the old saw about girls not knowing about money and figures is a myth. Girls start to outspend boys before puberty—and they manage to maintain this lead until death or an ugly credit manager, whichever comes first. Males are born with a closed fist. Girls are born with the left hand cramped in a position the size of an American Express card.

Whenever a girl sees a sign reading, "Sale, Going Out of Business, Liquidation," saliva begins to form in her mouth, the palms of her hands perspire and the pituitary gland says, "Go, Mama."

In the male, it is quite a different story. He has a gland that follows a muscle from the right arm down to the base of his billfold pocket. It's called "cheap."

Girls can slam a door louder, beg longer, turn tears on and off like a faucet and invented the term, "You don't trust me."

So much for "sugar and spice and everything nice" and "snips and snails and puppydog tails."

Erma Bombeck

On Being the Mother of Twins

I had always wanted to be a mother. In my youthful days, I could imagine running through a field of daisies with my children. My long hair would fall in great swirls about my face, radiant with motherhood. My children would look up adoringly at me, and the sun would shine warmly on us.

But I found real motherhood not like that at all. One day I took my four children to a field, even though I didn't have time to take the curlers out of my short stubborn hair.

One of the twins got stung by a bee and the other one picked poison ivy for me. The girls complained constantly about being thirsty. Just as the rain started, a man yelled, "Hey, get out of here. You're trespassing."

Why doesn't someone tell you what motherhood is really like? Why don't they tell you about mountains of crumbs that stick to high chairs and sticky spilled milk and sky-high temperatures. Why doesn't someone warn you about children who whine? Why don't they tell you how to get gum out of rugs and what to do when an apple gets flushed down the toilet?

Actually, I managed quite well as a mother with my first little girl. Julie was never sick, and anything suited her. She had regular checkups, ate a balanced diet, wore matching outfits and a pert ribbon in her hair, and always smelled of baby powder. I read to her by the hour. She could quote "Annabel Lee" in kindergarten.

Two years later a second daughter, Jennifer, arrived. Jennifer was a happy, contented baby, like her sister. Two little girls and a mother who had to hurry a bit but certainly believed that little girls were sugar and spice and everything nice.

But wouldn't a little boy be fun, I thought, as I saw my husband looking at boy babies or going out to play football with a neighbor's child. I wonder what little boys are like, I mused. So at the age of thirty-three, I was delighted to learn a baby was on the way. My husband and our girls were also thrilled.

I can still remember the kindly doctor looking at an x ray two months before my baby was due and holding up two fingers. I didn't know what he meant.

"Twins, Mrs. West, you're going to have twins!"

I expected girls again and had, back in my mind, the names Jessica and Johanna. But we quickly came up with the names Jonathan and Jeremy. I couldn't believe I had twin sons—or four children!

The trips to the pediatrician's office became so traumatic that I stopped going. There was always a little fellow who sat calmly by his mother's side glancing up at her lovingly. His shirt was buttoned, his pants zipped, socks matched, and both his shoes remained on and tied. His mother sighed to me, "I don't know what I'd do if I had two of little Albert."

As my twins, not quite a year old, crawled under people's chairs, onto strangers' laps and onto the window ledges, I thought grimly, *You should have five of him!*

Also in the waiting room was the mother with her firstborn. She became very protective as my sons made their way toward her baby. Her mother, husband and the maid discouraged my twins from coming close. When I gave Jon and Jeremy a whack on their bottoms, this young mother looked at me with an I'll-never-have-to-resort-to-that-sort-of-thing look.

As the twins got older, and I aged incredibly, I learned to move fast. Do I run after Jeremy as he heads for three empty bottles on my neighbor's carport or dash for Jon as he disappears into a storm drain? Should I catch the one getting into the bathtub fully clothed or go after the one pulling the hissing cat out from under the bed?

As the twins grew larger, they eventually covered every inch of the house looking for adventure. They turned over the television and removed its parts, broke out the glass in the French door, knocked out window screens and threw their clothes and toys out, climbed up inside the chimney, pulled down curtains and curtain rods, removed the heating ducts from the wall and finally turned over an old chest with each of them shut tightly in a drawer.

Some weeks were worse than others. One Tuesday afternoon, a railing outside the public library gave way and Jon fell eleven feet. That night, Jeremy knocked a tooth loose.

Wednesday, Jeremy learned to open the car door while I was driving. Saturday night, Jeremy leaped from the mantel and required five stitches in his head. Jon cried for days because he didn't have any stitches and finally consoled himself by drinking iodine.

Just before the boys were fifteen months old, Jeremy discovered how to get out of his bed. Then he freed Jon. This meant every day I dragged around the house like Frankenstein with a twin clinging to each leg.

The look in my eyes after a few days forced my husband to take drastic measures. He built a fence around the top of Jeremy's bed with chicken wire. When Jeremy climbed over the top of the fence and jumped to freedom,

Jerry built a top to the fence and put a lock on it.

We soon learned to ignore the looks on the faces of our friends when they saw Jeremy's bed for the first time. Actually, Jeremy seemed relieved to be confined, which proves what I have always believed: Children want discipline.

Jeremy's Sunday school teacher never did understand why he began placing a doll in a doll bed and then turning another bed over it, smiling with great satisfaction. I didn't tell her about Jeremy's bed.

Talking on the telephone was dangerous. My twins had become conditioned, and the sound of our phone ringing sent them looking for trouble.

One day as I talked on the phone (I had to communicate with people somehow), Jon came running to me looking funny, and holding his throat. We had just returned from the hospital that day. Jon's tonsils had been removed. Suddenly, I knew what his trouble was.

Surely, God must give mothers of twins extra abilities. Jon had found a nickel on my dresser and swallowed it.

I threw the phone down and grabbed Jon by the feet, shaking him and praying. Out came the nickel and his stitches didn't even bleed.

Friends almost stopped coming by. Our house was like a three-ring circus. I often stood by the window watching my friends going out to eat lunch together and felt an ache I thought I couldn't bear.

That same day a dear friend came by. I was so glad to see an adult, I could hardly stop talking or grinning. Our conversation was interrupted by loud crashes coming from the direction of the bathroom. Lord, help me ignore the noise and enjoy this friend who has come to see me.

Finally, as I continued to ignore the crashes, Jeremy brought me half of the top of the back of the toilet tank. He placed it in my lap, hoping to interrupt our conversation. I kept talking calmly, wiping the blood from his cut finger on my apron and cautioning him, "Don't bleed on the rug."

I almost never took the boys anywhere, but in desperation (it had rained for four days) we went to get a carton of soft drinks. My twins were wild with excitement.

I dressed Jon first. By the time I got to Jeremy, Jon stood inside the toilet bowl, laughing. I dressed Jon again and looked for Jeremy, only to find him standing out in the rain looking up with his mouth open.

Some mornings I awoke and prayed even before I opened my eyes: *Please, God, stay very close to me today. I don't even want to be a mother today. I just want to listen to silence and think my own thoughts, and brush my teeth without interruption.*

Going out was reduced to a jaunt to the garbage cans or a dash to the mailbox or the clothesline. One evening, however, I went to a dinner party with my husband. The children gathered around to watch me put on shoes and lipstick.

I guess the party was too much for me. I kept saying, "Look at all the big people." And I tried to cut the meat of the startled gentleman sitting next to me.

Sometimes I wonder how many miles I must have strolled Jon and Jeremy (mostly uphill) while Julie and Jennifer followed, constantly asking questions.

Many times I had no idea how I would do it one more day, or how I would even get through supper that night.

A little old lady who lived at the end of the street asked the same question. Many of my friends did. Even strangers sometimes quizzed me, "How do you manage?"

"I pray a lot," I told them. "I have to. I can't make it on my own. God helps me every day."

Marion Bond West

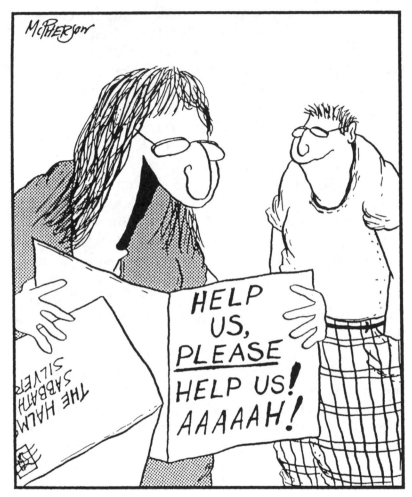

"Oh, wow! It's a birth announcement from the Fullersons! They just had twin boys!"

So You Want to Be a Mother?

I remember leaving the hospital . . . thinking wait, are they going to let me just walk off with him? I don't know beans about babies!

Anne Tyler

One of the biggest complaints about motherhood is the lack of training.

We all come to it armed only with a phone number for a diaper service, a Polaroid camera, a hotline to the pediatrician and innocence with a life span of fifteen minutes.

I have always felt that too much time was given before the birth, which is spent learning things like how to breathe in and out with your husband (I had my baby when they gave you a shot in the hip and you didn't wake up until the kid was ready to start school), and not enough time given to how to mother after the baby is born.

Motherhood is an art. And it is naive to send a mother into an arena for twenty years with a child and expect her to come out on top. Everything is in the child's favor. He's little. He's cute and he can turn tears on and off like a faucet.

There have always been schools for children. They spend anywhere from twelve to sixteen years of their lives in them, around other children who share the experience of being a child and how to combat it. They're in an academic atmosphere where they learn how to manipulate parents and get what they want from them. They bind together to form a children's network, where they pool ideas on how to get the car, how to get a bigger allowance and how to stay home when their parents go on a vacation. Their influence is felt throughout the world. Without contributing a dime, they have more ice cream parlors, recreation centers, playgrounds and amusement parks than any group could ever pull off.

They never pay full price for anything. How do they do it? They're clever and they're educated.

Some people think mothers should organize and form a union. I think education is the answer. If we only knew what to do and how to do it, we could survive.

It's only a dream now. But one of these days there will be a School for New Mothers that will elevate the profession to an academic level. What I wouldn't have given for a catalogue offering the following skills.

Creative Nagging 101: Learn from expert resource people how to make eye contact through a bathroom door, how to make a senior cry and how to make a child write you a check for bringing him into the world. More than 1,000 subjects guaranteed to make a child miserable for a lifetime. "Sit up straight or your spine will grow that way" and "Your aquarium just caught fire" are ordinary and boring. Creative Nagging gets you noticed! Child is furnished.

Seminar for Savers: No one dares call herself "Mother" until she has learned to save and horde. Squirreling away is not a congenital talent, as formerly believed. It can be learned. Find out where to store thirty pounds of twist ties from bread and cookie packages, old grade-school cards and boots with holes in the toe. Learn how to have a Christmas box for every occasion by snatching them from a person before they have taken the present out of it. Learn why hangers mate in dark closets and observe them as they reproduce. Mature language.

Investments and Returns from Your Children: Frank discussions on how to get your children to believe they owe you something. Each day mothers let opportunities for guilt slip through their fingers without even knowing it. The child who was ordered to "call when you get there" and doesn't, can be made to suffer for years. Find out how. Special attention is paid to Mother's Day and the child who once gave a forty-dollar cashmere sweater to a girl he had known only two weeks, while you, who have stomach muscles around your knees, received a set of bathroom soap in the shape of sea horses. Class size is limited.

Perfection: How to Get It and How to Convince Your Children You've Got It: The art of never making a mistake is crucial to motherhood. To be effective and to gain the respect she needs to function, a mother must have her children believe she has never engaged in sex, never made a bad decision, never caused her own mother a moment's anxiety and was never a child. Enrollment limited to those who have taken "The Madonna Face Mystique."

Legal Rights for Mothers: Know the law. Are you required to transport laundry that has been in the utility room longer than sixty days? Do you have the right to open a bedroom door with a skewer, or would this be considered illegal entry? Can you abandon a child along a public highway for kicking Daddy's seat for 600 miles? Are you liable for desertion if you move and don't tell your grown son where you are going? A panel of legal experts will discuss how binding is the loan of $600 from a two-month-old baby to his parents when there were no witnesses.

The History of Suspicion and Its Effects on Menopause: Due to popular demand, we are again offering this course for older mothers. How to tell when your child is telling the truth even after her nose has stopped growing. The following case histories of suspicion will be discussed: Did Marlene really drop a Bible on her foot, keeping her from getting to the post office and mailing the letter to her parents? Did twenty dollars really fall out of your purse and your son found it and kept it and didn't know how it got there? Was your son really in bed watching *Masterpiece Theatre* when he heard a racket and got up to discover 200 strangers having a party in the house and drinking all of Dad's beer? Physical examination required.

Threats and Promises: Four fun-filled sessions on how to use chilling threats and empty promises to intimidate your children for the rest of their lives. Graduates have nothing but praise for this course. One mother who told her daughter she would wet the bed if she played with matches said the kid was thirty-five before she would turn on a stove. Hurry. Enrollment limited.

Note: Guilt: The Gift that keeps giving has been canceled until an instructor can be found. Dr. Volland said his mother felt he had no business teaching others when he ignored his own mother.

Erma Bombeck

Growing Up Pains

My children are small, still lap-sized with many years ahead in my care. And yet, already I know, and I feel that one day, no matter how many diapers changed, bottles fed, books read, hands washed or faces kissed, it will never be quite long enough.

Jennifer Graham Billings

"Honey," my husband said when I was pregnant, "I promise. When the baby is born, I'll take over every night and every weekend." He lied.

My husband is a wonderful man. A wonderful father. He cried in the delivery room. He changes diapers without complaint. He doesn't even mind when our son throws up on him. But he works late and travels often. He has Friday-night business dinners, Sunday-morning meetings, and black-tie events to which wives are not invited. I'm a reasonable woman; I understand how weary he is. "I'm just not in the mood to give the baby a bath tonight," he says.

"I know what you mean," I say sympathetically. "I'm

not in the mood to give him dinner."

In my worst moments, I feel as if I have been sold a bill of goods. I was ambivalent about having children. I knew the radical changes it would impose: the limitations on my time, my independence, my work. And what bothered me most was that these changes would affect my day-to-day life, not my husband's. I'm not saying that being a father hasn't radically altered his view of the world and his place in it; I know that our son is the center of his universe. But it's just not the same for him. He still gets up every day, puts on grownup clothes and goes to an office where there are other reasonably mature adults making adult conversation. He goes out to lunch and doesn't have to cut up anyone's food. He has the luxury to stop after work for a drink, or to browse in a bookstore, knowing that it's okay because I've got him covered. He knows who's minding the store.

I have become that thing I dreaded most: a housewife. June Cleaver with an M.A., Donna Reed in running shoes. My mother. *Your* mother. And there are too many moments in my day when I wonder if I have the right credentials for this job. They license you for everything else except this, the hardest job of all. No one ever told me about the sheer tedium of doing the same Playskool puzzle twenty-two times in one hour, or using a toothbrush to scrape the mashed peas and calcified oatmeal out of the grout on the kitchen floor after every meal, while behind me my son gleefully empties the box of croissant crackers and dances on them.

Okay, okay. I'd read Erma Bombeck; I had an inkling of what I was in for. But I thought it would be different for me. After all, my husband read me poetry on our first date. For six years we were culture vultures, eagerly devouring literature, movies, art galleries, craft fairs and endless cups of espresso, talking with pent-up eagerness, in perfect accord. "When we have children, we'll read Piaget together," he said. Now, of course, while I'm consulting Penelope Leach or Dr. Spock, he's buried behind the *Wall Street Journal*. He has yet to pick up one book on child care.

This isn't the life I expected to have. This is only slightly mitigated by the fact that other women with small children tell me the same thing. I thought I'd be living in Manhattan, writing for *The New York Times*, giving wonderful intimate dinner parties where my cultured guests would discourse in sparkling fashion on politics and the arts. Instead, I live in a cozy colonial in Scarsdale, debate the relative merits of Gymboree over Tumbling Tots, swap recipes for home-made Play-Doh, and sponge Teddy Grahams off the living-room couch.

I'm mourning the loss of my options. I can always quit a job, sell a house, or even refuse a medical treatment, but I can never go back to being a non-parent. And with this, I have acquired a new, responsible persona. I have finally written a will, something that seemed so remote and unnecessary in my lighthearted twenties. I have appointed legal guardians for my child, and bought zero-coupon bonds as a hedge against his college tuition. But it is the smaller things that are more telling: I no longer jaywalk. Because now I know, as you never know when you are young, that something could happen to me. This scares me, not for my sake, but for my son's. And despite the fact that I have given up freedom, choices and the pleasure of hav-ing an uninterrupted conversation with another adult dur-ing daylight hours, the truth is that I need my child as much as he needs me. Life without him is unimaginable. Before I became a mother, there were three things that no one could have told me: how much labor would hurt; how tedious life with a toddler could be; and how passionately I would love my child.

Liane Kupferberg Carter

Loving Adam

I didn't think it would be that way. When I first learned my baby would be born with Down's syndrome, I was devastated. My husband, John and I are Harvard alumni who once held intelligence as the prize above all others. I remember passing a homeless man who looked at my abdomen and said, "Congratulations, Mama!" *If he only knew,* I thought bitterly.

Now the memory makes me smile. Maybe that man did know. Maybe he was an angel in disguise who could have told me, "Your little boy may not look like what you asked for, or be able to perform all the tricks. But he will light up your life."

Something in my son always manages to see past the outward ordinariness of a thing to any magic it may hold inside. One Christmas, for instance, he fished around under the tree until he found a package with his name on it. It was from my friend Annette, his honorary aunt. He tore the paper off the package, holding his breath, and found batteries. An eight-pack of D's, still encased in plastic.

"Oh, honey," I said, "that's not the real present." I was going to say that the batteries were meant to go in the big, noisy, light-up gun that I knew Annette was giving him, which lay still wrapped under the tree. But Adam was staring at those batteries, his mouth open in astonished ecstasy. "Oh, wow!" he said. "Mom, look! Batteries!" (It actually sounded more like "Mom, 'ook! Aggabies!" but the message was clear). Before his father, sisters Katie and Lizzie, or I could divert his attention to any other gift, Adam leapt to his feet and began running around the house, locating every appliance, tool and toy that ran on batteries. The whole time, he babbled excitedly about all the things he could do with this fabulous, fabulous gift.

As we watched, it began to occur to all of us "normal" people that batteries really were a pretty darn good Christmas present. They didn't look like much on the face of it, but think what they could do! Put them in place, and inanimate objects suddenly came to life, moving, talking, singing, lighting up the room.

Adam also has a way of putting my worries into proper perspective. When he was three years old, he could not speak. It was terribly frustrating for him, and it just plain broke my heart. I worked with him for hours, doing the exercises the speech therapists had taught me, but had no success whatsoever. I had to face it: Adam couldn't talk. Not at all. One day, after hours of unsuccessful therapy, I hit a low point. I took my three children to the grocery store and offered them all bribes to keep quiet—I was too tired to enforce discipline any other way. Each could pick out a treat from the candy stands next to the checkout counter.

Katie chose a roll of Life Savers and Lizzie a chocolate bar. Adam went over to a basket of red rosebuds and pulled one out. "This is what you want?" I asked incredulously. He nodded. "Honey, this isn't candy," I said, putting it back and turning him toward the rows of sweets. "Don't you want candy?"

He shook his small head, walked back to the bucket, picked out the rose and put it on the counter. I was baffled, but paid for it. Adam took it gravely and held the flower with both hands all the way home. When we got there, I was immediately engrossed in putting away the groceries and forgot all about his strange request.

The next morning I awoke to find sunlight streaming through my bedroom window. John had already left for the day, and I heard quiet babbling coming from Lizzie's room.

As I yawned and stretched, I could hear Adam's small feet padding down the hall toward my room. He appeared at the door with the rose. Walking over to the bed, he held out the flower and said in a clear, calm voice, "Here." Then he turned around, his little blue pajamas dragging a bit on the floor, and padded out.

Another one of my biggest fears had been that Adam would never learn to read or write. From the time he started preschool, John and I kept running through the alphabet with him, repeating each letter. But Adam never recognized the letters on his own. By the time he was six, I was ready to give up.

Then one day, John held up a plastic letter *e* and sounded out, *Ee*. Adam suddenly perked up and said, "Wisbef"—his way of pronouncing his sister Elizabeth's name. John and I stayed home from work to celebrate.

We discovered that Adam's learning capacity went way beyond anything we had expected—as long as it related directly to someone he cared about. He had no interest in "*E* is for egg," but *E* for Elizabeth, *G* for Grandpa, *K* for Katie, *M* for Mom—now that was crucial information. Another time Adam came home to tell me about the new boy in his class who had become his friend. When I couldn't understand his pronunciation of the boy's name, Adam grabbed a pencil in his stubby little boy fingers and wrote "Miguel Fernando de la Hoya" on a piece of paper that, needless to say, I intend to frame. If I ever need a dose of Adam and he isn't around, I'll look at the clumsily written name and remember what it is like to tap into an intelligence powered exclusively by love.

Living with Adam, loving Adam, has had moments of pain and disappointment, but mostly with people who look at my son and see only the deformity of their own perceptions instead of the beauty before their eyes. More and more, I feel this pain, not for my son but for the people who are too blind to see him. Once I was blind, but Adam has given me sight. It is impossible to look at his smile and not smile back.

Albert Einstein once said that the single most important decision any of us will ever make is whether or not to believe the universe is friendly. When Adam grins, it's clear he has made that decision affirmatively. Now I rely on my amazing little boy to be my guide in this new world where joy is commonplace, Harvard academics are the slow learners and children with Down's syndrome the master teachers.

Martha Beck

Love Letters to My Daughter

It was a balmy summer day in late July. I had been feeling rather queasy and nauseated, so I decided to see my doctor. "Mrs. Hayes, I'm happy to tell you that you are ten weeks pregnant," my doctor announced. I couldn't believe my ears. It was a dream come true.

My husband and I were young and had been married for only a year. We were working hard to build a happy life together. The news that we were expecting a baby was exciting and scary.

In my youthful enthusiasm I decided to write "love letters" to our baby to express my feelings of expectancy and joy. Little did I know just how valuable those love letters would be in the years to come.

> August 1971: *Oh, my darling baby, can you feel the love I have for you while you are so small and living in the quiet world inside my body? Your daddy and I want the world to be perfect for you with no hate, no wars, no pollution. I can't wait to hold you in my arms in just six months! I love you, and Daddy loves you but he can't feel you yet.*

September 1971: I am four months pregnant and am feeling better. I can tell you are growing, and I hope you are well and comfortable. I've been taking vitamins and eating healthy foods for you. Thank goodness my morning sickness is gone. I think about you all the time.

October 1971: Oh, these melancholy moods. I cry so often over so little. Sometimes I feel very alone, and then I remember you are growing inside of me. I feel you stirring, now tumbling and turning and pushing. It's never the same. Your movements always bring me so much joy!

November 1971: I am feeling much better now that my fatigue and nausea have passed. The intense heat of summer is over. The weather is lovely, crisp and breezy. I feel your movements often now. Constant punching and kicking. What elation to know you are alive and well. Last week Daddy and I heard your strong heartbeat at the doctor's office.

February 2, 1972 at 11:06 P.M.: You were born! We named you Sasha. It was a long, hard twenty-two hour labor, and your daddy helped me relax and stay calm. We are so happy to see you, to hold you, and to greet you. Welcome, our firstborn child. We love you so much!

Sasha was soon one year old and cautiously toddling all over the house. Then she was riding ponies and swinging in the sunshine at the park. Our little blue-eyed beauty entered kindergarten and grew into a bright and strong-willed little girl. The years passed so quickly that my husband and I joked that we put our five-year-old daughter to bed one night and she woke up the next morning as a teenager.

Those few years of adolescence and rebellion were not easy. There were times my beautiful yet angry teenage would dig her feet into the ground and yell. "You never loved me! You don't care about me or want me to be happy!"

Her harsh words cut at my heart. After one of my daughter's angry outbursts, I suddenly remembered the little box of love letters tucked away in my bedroom closet. I found them and quietly placed them on her bed, hoping she would read them. A few days later, she appeared before me with tears in her eyes.

"Mom, I never knew just how much you truly loved me—even before I was born!" she said. "How could you love me without knowing me? You loved me unconditionally!" That very precious moment became a bond of unity that still exists between us today because of those dusty old love letters.

Judith Hayes

Guilt-Free Parenting

There are one hundred and fifty-two distinctly different ways of holding a baby—and all are right.

Heywood Broun

There are books out there touting theories of every aspect of parenthood, many of them conflicting (and many of them bestsellers!). This overabundance of advice is precisely why I have decided to add my own theory to the mix.

It is simply this: The best parenting is Guilt-Free Parenting.

In other words: Do the research, listen to the opinions, then choose to do exactly what works for you, your baby and your family, and don't let anyone make you feel guilty about it!

Even if your baby isn't born yet, you have probably been acquainted with the "good parenting by guilt" conundrum. In other words, "There is one right way to raise your child and if you don't do it this correct way, your child will doubtless grow up to saw off his own shotguns." Followed shortly by, "Society as a whole has not parented correctly and that's why we're in the trouble we're in!" And you start feeling guilty pre-labor because you just know you're going to mess up. Somehow.

Well, you know what? You are. Everybody does. Kids survive. Become happy, productive members of society even. I can't tell you how many great moms I know who are driven by guilt: They stay home; they don't stay home. They allow television; they don't allow television. They believe in the Family Bed; they're strict Ferberians. Whichever you choose, you feel like society is coming down hard on your chosen side.

Well, it shouldn't. And even if it does, you have permission not to care.

Being a mom is wonderful, and it is tough. So wonderful and so tough that we all need to stick together and applaud each other like mad, not trounce around trying to find someone who's doing it worse than we are to make ourselves feel better.

Let me give you some specific cases in point.

I am a good mom. I adore my children and they, thankfully, adore me. (And will, I tell myself, even when they'll turn fifteen and pierce something not yet thought of and threaten to leave home because their dad and I will never understand. Been there, threatened that.)

But let me be more precise. I am a good not-full-time mom. Yes, I work outside the home (well, actually I work inside the home and send my children to play outside the home) and I have, part time, since each of my two children was six weeks old. I do it partly because I love my work and partly because the family can use the money. But I do it mostly because I'm a better mom that way. When I'm alone with my two adorable children twenty-four hours a day, they make me crazy. And I make them crazy in return. When I am away from them even a few hours, we are thrilled to see each other and have touching, hug-filled reunions. Yes, I was there to hear their first words, see their first steps, watch them eat their first Play-Doh. Even if you're away forty hours a week, that leaves 128 at home. True, some of those remaining hours are at night, but anyone who thinks significant parenting doesn't happen at night has never had a sick or frightened child.

I come by this honestly. My mom, who is a great mother, was also a teacher. When she was working, she was much happier, and so were we. As they say, When Mama ain't happy, ain't nobody happy.

Perhaps the most important thing I learned in my college sociology class was that God made people tribal animals, and we lived as such for centuries. This whole nuclear family thing—the idea that two people, a husband and wife, can fulfill every job for nurture and survival of the family themselves—is a fairly recent, very American development. Think about it. In the olden days (and still, in some places in the world), the extended family or village pooled its resources. The women who were talented in cooking spent their days with their like-minded sisters in the kitchens. The men who were skilled farmers hoed; those who had hunting skills hunted, those who could tailor, tailored. Aunts, sisters and cousins joined together to care for the kids. That gave you three or four women friends to chat with while you were cooking or cleaning or spinning or watching the children. (And your best friends were the women. This idea that your husband had to be your best friend as well as your mate is pretty recent, also. Being a good provider and bearer of good genes used to do it.)

Now, we expect two people to have every single skill between them. We are such an individualistic society that we send two parents (or, God bless them, one parent) and children into their own dwelling and shut them in, expecting all the cooking, cleaning, wage-earning, food-gathering, child-caring, money-tending chores to be done between them, even if they are not skilled in many of these areas. It is a very rare mom who can be locked in a house with only short people for twenty-four hours a day and not go nuts.

Now, I am not saying moms should immediately go out and work. Far from it! I think God gave some women the gift of mothering. There are some women who can be with children thirty-six hours a day and retire to their rooms worn out but happy. These women should immediately be named National Treasures, and we should offer them six-figure salaries to watch after our children. Seriously.

Stay-at-home moms, you have my complete awe and respect. What you are doing is absolutely wonderful. And, not only that, you should have full permission to moan and complain when you need to and not have anyone think less of you for it. One of the main rules of Guilt-Free Parenting is that moms shouldn't have to pretend their choice is perfect and defend it to the death. It's hard to be a stay-at-home mom. It's hard to be a working mom. And you should know moms who have made the other choice are as exhausted and often perplexed as you are.

Working moms, enjoy your work, enjoy your kids. Does it bother me one bit that my kids call my child care provider Mommy Sara and me Mommy Mommy? Not one bit. They can never have too much love. Nor does it bother me when one of the kids comes home from Mommy Sara's bumped and bruised from sledding or cat-scratched. (This usually happens just before a major holiday or portrait sitting.) I can't expect more of Mommy Sara than I do of myself. Nor do I mind that she seems to think of Cheerios as a food group. I stuff enough salmon and broccoli into my kids to make up for it. (Our other family-care provider is a vegetarian nutritionist, so I think together they balance each other out.)

(Plus, frankly, at college graduation, will they even remember Mommy Sara? Who knows? But I'll sure be there, God willing, having footed the bill!)

As far as other parenting choices: Breast feeding is great. If you can't do it for whatever reason, your child will survive—all of us born in the 1950s did.

And how about co-sleeping? That one will get a sprightly conversation going. We have one set of friends who believe mightily in the Family Bed; when I first met their two-year-old son, he had never spent the night in a bed without one or both of his parents. (He looked healthy and well adjusted. They looked exhausted.) We have other friends who believe completely in the Dr. Ferber's Method of teaching your child to be self-sufficient and sleep through the night in his or her own bed practically from the time he or she is born. Us? My husband and I are, once again, middle-of-the-roaders. My two-year-old daughter has just moved to a "big girl bed" and she comes padding in some nights when she's scared. I love it. I love her little body close to mine and her shallow breath. (I love thinking that would-be kidnappers would have to find her first, then get past me to get her.) I also know her five-year-old brother did the same thing at two and now Santa and the Tooth Fairy singing a rock duet couldn't wake him from his own bed.

And the whole discussion of television. We have friends who let their four-year-old watch late night TV, and other friends who have chosen not to own a set. Frankly, I see the television simply as a medium which is neither good nor bad in itself; it's the particular show that must be judged. (And, good news, there are some great kids shows these days! Check out *Arthur* and *Blue's Clues* for starters

Little Bear also encourages mother-worship.) To our friends who have chosen not to own a set (and tried to make me feel guilty for choosing differently), I said, "We paid extra for an Off Button. And we use it."

But the main tenet of this Guilt-Free Parenting is to enjoy your children. Don't be so worried about how to do it right that you don't trust your instincts. Have fun together.

Show them what they can do more often than telling them what they can't. Take a good parenting class—there's no use reinventing the wheel. Put together an extended community however and whenever you can. Never take anything a two-year-old says or does personally.

Laugh a lot.

Are my kids the best-behaved kids in America? Uh, no. (Do we try valiantly to teach them manners? You bet.) Could they speak French at three? Don't think so. Potty-trained overnight? Nope.

But a year ago I overheard our handyman say to his wife, "Those are the happiest darn kids I've ever seen!"

You'll have those moments too. When the choices you've made feel right. God bless you!

Together we soldier on.

Sharon Linnéa

More Chicken Soup?

Many of the stories and poems you have read in this book were submitted by readers like you who had read earlier *Chicken Soup for the Soul* books. We are planning to publish new *Chicken Soup for the Soul* books every year. We invite you to contribute a story to one of these future volumes.

Stories may be up to 1,200 words and must uplift or inspire. You may submit an original piece or something you clip out of the local newspaper, a magazine, a church bulletin or a company newsletter. It could also be your favorite quotation you've put on your refrigerator door or a personal experience that has touched you deeply.

To obtain a copy of our submission guidelines and a listing of upcoming *Chicken Soup* books, please write, fax or check our Web sites.

Chicken Soup for the *(Specify Which Edition)* Soul
P.O. Box 30880 • Santa Barbara, CA 93130
fax: 805-563-2945
To e-mail or visit our Web site:
www.chickensoup.com

You can also visit the *Chicken Soup for the Soul* site on America Online at keyword: *chickensoup*.

Just send a copy of your stories and other pieces, indicating which edition they are for, to any of the above addresses. We will be sure that both you and the author are credited for your submission.

For information about speaking engagements, other books, audiotapes, workshops and training programs, please contact any of the authors directly.

Passing It On!

It has become a tradition to donate a portion of the net profits of every *Chicken Soup for the Soul* book to several charities related to the theme of the book. Past recipients have included the American Red Cross, The Wellness Community, the Breast Cancer Research Foundation, the National Arbor Association, the American Association of University Women Educational Foundation, and Literacy Volunteers of America.

We will select several worthy charities that will receive a portion of the proceeds from this book. With your cooperation, it's our hope to truly change lives, one book at a time.

Who Is Jack Canfield?

Jack Canfield is one of America's leading experts in the development of human potential and personal effectiveness throughout the life span. He is both a dynamic, entertaining speaker and a highly sought-after trainer. Jack has a wonderful ability to inform and inspire audiences toward increased levels of self-esteem and peak performance at every stage of life.

He is the author and narrator of several bestselling audio- and videocassette programs, including *Self-Esteem and Peak Performance, How to Build High Self-Esteem, Self-Esteem in the Classroom* and *Chicken Soup for the Soul—Live.* He is regularly seen on television shows such as *Good Morning America, 20/20* and *NBC Nightly News.* Jack has co-authored numerous books, including the *Chicken Soup for the Soul* series, *Dare to Win* and *The Aladdin Factor* (all with Mark Victor Hansen), *100 Ways to Build Self-Concept in the Classroom* (with Harold C. Wells), *101 Ways to Develop Student Self-Esteem and Responsibility* (with Frank Siccone) and *Heart at Work* (with Jacqueline Miller).

Jack is a regularly featured speaker for professional associations, school districts, government agencies, churches, hospitals, sales organizations and corporations. His clients have included the American Dental Association, the American Management Association, AT&T, Campbell Soup, Clairol, Domino's Pizza, GE, ITT, Hartford Insurance, Johnson & Johnson, the Million Dollar Roundtable, NCR, New England Telephone, Re/Max, Scott Paper, TRW and Virgin Records.

Jack conducts an annual eight-day Training of Trainers program in the areas of self-esteem and peak performance. It attracts educators, counselors, parenting trainers, corporate trainers, professional speakers, ministers and others interested in developing their speaking and seminar-leading skills.

For further information about Jack's books, tapes and training programs, or to schedule him for a presentation, please contact:

Self-Esteem Seminars
P. O. Box 30880
Santa Barbara, CA 93130
Phone: 805-563-2935
Fax: 805-563-2945
Web site: *http://www.chickensoup.com*

Who Is Mark Victor Hansen?

Mark Victor Hansen is a professional speaker who, in the last twenty years, has made over four thousand presentations to more than two million people in thirty-two countries. His presentations cover sales excellence and strategies; personal empowerment and development regardless of stages of life; and how to triple your income and double your time off.

Mark has spent a lifetime dedicated to his mission of making a profound and positive difference in people's lives. Throughout his career, he has inspired hundreds of thousands of people to create a more powerful and purposeful future for themselves while stimulating the sale of billions of dollars worth of goods and services.

Mark is a prolific writer and has authored *Future Diary, How to Achieve Total Prosperity* and *The Miracle of Tithing.* He is coauthor of the *Chicken Soup for the Soul* series, *Dare to Win* and *The Aladdin Factor* (all with Jack Canfield), *The Master Motivator* (with Joe Batten) and *Out of the Blue* (with Barbara Nichols).

Mark has also produced a complete library of personal empowerment audio- and videocassette programs that have enabled his listeners to recognize and use their innate abilities in their business and personal lives. His message has made him a popular television and radio personality, with appearances on ABC, NBC, CBS, HBO, PBS and CNN. He has also appeared on the cover of numerous magazines, including *Success, Entrepreneur* and *Changes.*

Mark is a big man with a heart and spirit to match—an inspiration to people of all ages who seek to better themselves.

For further information about Mark write:

MVH & Associates
P. O. Box 7665
Newport Beach, CA 92658
Phone: 714-759-9304 or 800-433-2314
Fax: 714-722-6912
Web site: *http://www.chickensoup.com*

Who Is Patty Aubery?

Patty Aubery is the vice president of The Canfield Training Group and Self-Esteem Seminars, Inc. Patty came to work for Jack Canfield in 1989, when Jack still ran his organization out of his house in Pacific Palisades. Patty has been working with Jack since the birth of *Chicken Soup for the Soul* and can remember the days of struggling to market the book. Patty says, "I can remember sitting at flea markets in 100 degree weather trying to sell the book and people would stop, look and walk to the next booth! They thought I was crazy. Everyone said I was wasting my time. And now here I am. Fourteen million copies have been sold of the first eleven books, and I have coauthored two of the books in the *Chicken Soup* series!"

Patty is the coauthor of *Chicken Soup for the Surviving Soul: 101 Stories of Courage and Inspiration from Those Who Have Survived Cancer.* She has been a guest on over fifty local and nationally syndicated radio shows.

Patty is married to Jeff Aubery, and together they have two sons. Patty and her family reside in Santa Barbara, California, and can be reached at The Canfield Training Group, P.O. Box 30880, Santa Barbara, CA 93130, or by calling 805-563-2935, or faxing 805-563-2945.

Who Is Nancy Mitchell?

Nancy Mitchell is the director of copyrights and permissions for the *Chicken Soup for the Soul* series. She graduated from Arizona State University in May of 1994 with a B.S. in Nursing. After graduation Nancy worked at Good Samaritan Regional Medical Center in Phoenix, Arizona, in the Cardiovascular Intensive Care Unit. Four months after graduation, Nancy moved back to her native town of Los Angeles and became involved with the *Chicken Soup* series. Nancy's intentions were to help finish *A 2nd Helping of Chicken Soup for the Soul* and then return to nursing. However, in December of that year, she was asked to continue on full time at The Canfield Group. Nancy put nursing on hold and became the director of publishing, working closely with Jack and Mark on all *Chicken Soup for the Soul* projects.

Nancy says that what she is most thankful for right now is her move back to Los Angeles. "If I hadn't moved back to California, I wouldn't have had the chance to be there for my mom during her bout with breast cancer." Out of that struggle Nancy coauthored *Chicken Soup for the Surviving Soul: 101 Stories of Courage and Inspiration from Those Who Have Survived Cancer.* Little did she know that the book would become her own inspiration when her dad was diagnosed with prostate cancer in 1999.

Nancy also coauthored *Chicken Soup for the Christian Family Soul* and will coauthor the upcoming *Chicken Soup for the Nurse's Soul.* Nancy resides in Santa Barbara with her golden retriever, Kona.

Reach her at: The Canfield Group, P.O. Box 30880, Santa Barbara, CA 93130, or by calling 805-563-2935, or faxing 805-563-2945, or via e-mail at *www.chickensoup.com.*

Contributors

Several of the stories in this book were taken from previously published sources, such as books, magazines and newspapers. These sources are acknowledged in the permissions section. However, most of the stories were written by humorists, comedians, professional speakers and workshop presenters. If you would like to contact them for information on their books, audiotapes and videotapes, seminars and workshops, you can reach them at the addresses and phone numbers provided below.

The remainder of the stories were submitted by readers of our previous *Chicken Soup for the Soul* books who responded to our requests for stories. We have also included information about them.

Cynthia Anderson lives in Lexington, Massachusetts, with her family, and teaches at Boston University. Her essays and short stories have appeared in *House Beautiful, Redbook, Yankee, The North American Review, Literal Latte* and others. Contact her at: *cbawrite3@aol.com*.

Antoinette Bosco was formerly executive editor of the *Litchfield County Times*.

Debra Ayers Brown is Meredith's mom and director of marketing of Savannah Tech. She graduated magna cum laude from the University of Georgia and has a master's of business administration. She is a member of the Southeastern Writers' Association. Her inspirational stories have been included in *Guideposts* and in the *Chocolate* series.

Elizabeth Butera was born in Rochester, New York, where she still lives today. She enjoys playing volleyball, camping, decorating cakes and writing poetry. Elizabeth has a large wonderful family and many caring friends, all of whom she is deeply grateful for. Her favorite thing to do is travel to the ocean.

Jan Butsch is an Atlanta native, raising two children. She has taught parenting classes and has written a parenting column since 1995, for which she has received three finalist awards from the Society of Professional Journalists. She is a graduate of the University of Virginia and is the editor at Schroder Publishing in Atlanta.

Patricia K. Cameransi was born in Eugene, Oregon, and graduated from Oregon State University with a degree in communications. After graduation she moved to Washington, D.C., and worked in public relations and government. For the past ten years, Patricia was a marketing director in the architectural/engineering industry. She currently resides in Florence, South Carolina, with her husband and son.

Bill Canty's cartoons have appeared in many national magazines including the *Saturday Evening Post, Good Housekeeping, Better Homes and Gardens, Woman's World, National Review* and *Medical Economics*. His syndicated feature *All About Town* runs in thirty-five newspapers. Bill can be reached at P.O. Box 1053, S. Wellfleet, MA 02663. Phone and fax: 508-349-7549. He can be reached by e-mail at: *wcanty@mediaone.net* or visit his Web site at *www.reuben.org/Canty*.

Dave Carpenter has been a full-time cartoonist since 1981. His work has appeared in a number of publications including *Harvard Business Review, Barron's, Wall Street Journal, Reader's Digest, USA Weekend, Saturday Evening Post, Better Homes and Gardens, Good Housekeeping* and several *Chicken Soup for the Soul* books. Dave can be reached at P.O. Box 520, Emmetsburg, IA 50536.

Jacqueline Carrico is a forty-two-year-old wife, mother and nurse. She and her husband have a wonderful fourteen-year-old son. Jacqueline believes being his mother is her true job in life. This is her first submission for publication.

Liane Kupferberg Carter is a freelance writer whose work has appeared in the *New York Times Syndicate, McCall's, Parents, Child, Glamour, Cosmopolitan, New Parent* and *Newsday*. She lives in New York with her family, where she is a community activist for children with special needs. Reach her at *Lcarter@cloud9.net*.

Susanna Burkett Chenoweth has enjoyed working in many areas of nursing over the years, but has always considered her most rewarding role to be Mom. Blessed with two daughters, both grown, she lives in Danville, Indiana, with Roy, her husband of twenty-four years. She has been previously published in religious and children's magazines.

Robin Clifton lives in New Hope, Minnesota, with her husband, Jerry, and their four children. She grew up in the Minnesota river town of Red Wing, where her story takes place. The proud grandparents (her parents), Bob and Genene Gordish, still live there today.

Helen Colella is a wife, mother, former teacher, and freelance writer. She lives in Colorado with her family. She enjoys reading, traveling and being with her family and friends. And after twenty years, still marvels at the beautiful and majestic scenery of the Rocky Mountains.

Ron Coleman began cartooning while in junior high school, selling his first cartoon at age fourteen. He is published in hundreds of publications and is the creator of two cartoon Web sites: *http://cartoonfactory.com* and *http://belvedere-comics.com*. Currently he is involved in the creation of Flash animation projects for the Internet.

John Conklin is thirteen years old and attends Owosso Middle School. He lives with his mother and two brothers; David who is ten, and Michael, who is nine years old. John wrote this poem in school when his mother was pregnant. He saw Michael during an ultrasound and got pictures of him while he was in his mother's womb.

Kristen Cook works as a reporter in Tucson, Arizona. To prepare for impending parenthood, she and her husband practiced diapering and burping their two Australian shepherds. And happily, she did finally stop throwing up.

Scott Cramer lives near Boston with his wife and two daughters. He works as an Internet communications manager. He also writes general and travel freelance articles and children's picture books. He recently designed and is ready to market a kid's board game, Alley Cats. He can be reached at *cramer@crouton.com.*

Sharon Crismon, a wife and mother, resides in Dorr, Michigan. She enjoys spending time with family and friends. Sharon lost her dad on March 8, 1977. Her daughter, Samantha, was born December 16, 1998. Without words being said, these two touched so many lives. Sharon felt a strong need to tell her story, to give the world faith in miracles.

Eileen Davis is a writer of poetry, short stories and novels. She has completed a collection of reflective, short stories titled "Of Me I Sing," and a novel *Yesterday I Woke Up Dead.* Eileen is president and CEO of two wholesale food and distribution corporations and is presently working on a collection of business-related short stories and a cookbook.

Phyllis DeMarco is the mother of two great boys and a freelance writer with short stories published in *The Star, True Love* and *True Story. The Staten Island Advance* and *Staten Island Parent Magazine* have published her articles and two of her stories were recited by the S.I. Shakespearean Theater Company.

John Drescher was born and raised near Lancaster, Pennsylvania. He is married to Betty Keener and they are the parents of five grown children. He has authored twenty-eight books among which are *Seven Things Children Need, If I Were Starting My Family Again, Now Is the Time to Love, Spirit Fruit, When You Think You Are in Love, Meditations for the Newly Married, Why I Am a Conscientious Objector* and *If I Were Starting Our Marriage Again.* John has written for more than 100 different magazines and journals. His books have appeared in ten different languages. He has spoken at numerous conventions, retreats, and seminars—particularly in the area of family life.

Martine Ehrenclou has a four-year-old daughter and an eighteen-year-old stepson. She survived being a new mother and has gone back to graduate school to finish her masters in psychology at Pepperdine University, Los Angeles. She is a freelance writer and is at work finishing her first novel.

Lori Elmore-Moon is forty-two years old and married to Marcus Moon. The reside in Burleson, Texas, with their two sons from a previous marria

David Joshua Elmore and Nicholas Wayne Elmore. Lori currently works as a freelance journalist/writer, photographer and artist. She has previously been employed as an editor in the newspaper industry.

Jackie Fleming is a native Californian and her age is somewhere between forty and death. She has three grown sons and, at last count, ten grandchildren. Her hobby is traveling the world by freighter. Jackie's publishing credits are mostly in newspapers, since she wrote a column for two weekly publications for six years.

Patricia Franklin is a very happily married mother of five; three boys and two girls. She resides in West Virginia with her husband and three youngest children. She is very proud to share the story of her husband's bravery as they prepared for the birth of their third child.

Allison Yates Gaskins is the coauthor with her mother, Susan Yates, of *Thanks, Mom, for Everything,* from which this excerpt was taken. She also coauthored *Thanks, Dad, for Everything* and *Tightening the Knot.* She currently lives in Springfield, Virginia, with her husband and their two young children.

Dianne Gill is a freelance writer for *Woman's World* and *First Magazine for Women.* She has two grown children and resides in Long Island, New York, with her husband, Steve. Her hobbies are reading, gardening and photography.

Randy Glasbergen is one of America's most widely and frequently published cartoonists. More than 25,000 of his cartoons have been published by *Funny Times, Glamour,* Hallmark Cards, *Woman's World,* America Online, *Good Housekeeping* and many others. His daily comic panel *The Better Half* is syndicated worldwide by King Feature Syndicate. Randy is also the author of many cartoon books, including *Oh Baby!,* a collection of cartoons for new parents. You can find more of Randy's cartoons online at *www.glasbergen.com.*

Gilbert Goodman was born Gilbert Jay Goodman in Lansing, Michigan, on May 12, 1935. He grew up in Michigan and in 1954 joined the Marine Corps and came to California. He married Joan Crass in 1957, and has held careers with Pacific Telephone and IBM. He retired in 1996 and now spends his time traveling and enjoying his four grandchildren.

Debbie Graziano lives in the Chicago area with her husband and two wonderful children. She was born and raised there but spent many years on the West Coast. She is a second grade teacher and in her spare time she loves to have fun with her sons.

Stephen Harrigan is a contributing editor to the *Texas Monthly* and a frequent contributor to many other magazines. He is the author of six books, the most recent of which is *The Gates of the Alamo* (Alfred A. Knopf).

Jdith Hayes was born in Culver City, California, in 1949 and has been married to Michael since 1970. Judith and Michael have two daughters, Sarah, a registered nurse and Annabelle, a professional make-up artist. Judith was a Bradley childbirth instructor for eighteen years and taught childbirth classes at Northridge Hospital for thirteen years. She was also the program director for a home for unwed mothers. Judith coauthored *Create in Me a Clean Heart,* published by Thomas Nelson Books in 1995. Judith spends her time freelance writing.

Caroline Castle Hicks is a former contributor whose work also appears in *A Second Chicken Soup for the Woman's Soul.* A former high school English and humanities teacher, she is now a stay-at-home mom, freelance writer, poet and frequent public radio commentator. She lives just outside of Charlotte, North Carolina, with her husband, Dana, and their two children, Mariclaire and Ian. Her e-mail address is *dhicks1@compuserve.com.*

Barbara Hoffman never quite got over "Harriet the Spy" and became a newspaper reporter. These days, she roams New York City with her pen and pad. Occasionally, her son Sam joins her. Happily, he's become a lot more tactful.

Bunny Hoest is one of the most widely read cartoonists today, reaching nearly 200 million readers every week. She has produced *The Lockhorns, Agatha Crum, What a Guy!* and *Hunny Bunny's Short Tale,* distributed internationally by King Features; *Laugh Parade* featuring Howard Huge for Parade, seen by more than 80 million people every Sunday; and *Bumper Snickers* for the *National Enquirer,* with a circulation above seven million. This dynamic and versatile talent has twenty-five bestselling anthologies and a host of exciting new projects in the works, including a *Lockhorns* TV pilot and a *Howard Huge* animated feature in development with Merv Griffin Entertainment.

Melanie L. Huber was born off the coast of Oregon. Her family moved to the foothills of the Rocky Mountains in Idaho where she spent most of her childhood. Melanie went on to college in Kentucky after high school. She met her husband at Denny's Restaurant where she was a waitress and he a cook. When her husband finished college, they moved to West Virginia. They have four children: Halee, Ashley, Benjamin and Analee. Melanie is a homeschooling mom whose inspiration for writing comes from her children.

Patsy Hughes was born to Eugene G. and Deborah L. Gilliam, and is an avid reader of the *Chicken Soup for the Soul* book series. She balances her life between being a single mother of two teenaged boys, Daniel and Jeremy, and a full-time legal assistant to Attorney Robert G. Robinson. Patricia has been an active member of her community.

Cynthia Hummel is a professional freelance writer living in Strasburg, Pennsylvania, with her husband, Kirk and adopted son, Joshua. She writes for newspapers and magazines on a variety of subjects, including adoption. Cynthia's adoption stories focus on educating others about the challenges and rewards of adoption.

Francoise Inman was born in Madagascar and raised in France, Belgium and the United States. She is the mother of four boys, ages seven, four and a half, two and a newborn. She may be reached at *Inmancorp@n2mail.com.*

Antionette Ishmael is a sixth-grade teacher at Visitation School in Kansas City, Missouri. She was the 1997 recipient of The Excellence in Teaching Award. She enjoys writing and coaching, but most of all, she loves being the wife of Phil and the mom of Patrick, Anthony and Dominic. You may contact Antionette by email at *aishmael@school.visitation.org.*

Kelli S. Jones is a freelance writer, editor and pastor's wife living in Atlanta, Georgia. She shares her home with her husband Jeff and sons, Matt and Dan. Her latest project is entitled, "Everything You Always Wanted to Know About Your Pastor But Couldn't Dig Up." E-mail her at *paragonedit@mindspring.com.*

Kyle Louise Jossi is a nurse in a busy ER in suburban Maryland. She also does trauma reenactments for high school students to illustrate the dangers of drinking and driving. She has two wonderful daughters, Kiersten and Meredith, who are proof that raising teenagers can be fun. She enjoys horseback riding, writing and spending time with her husband, David.

Anna Maria Junus is a homemaker and writer residing with her husband and seven children in Alberta, Canada. She is the author of several unpublished children's books and has a poetry corner on the *family.com* Web site. She is currently working on a youth novel and has plans for several more, however she has no plans for more children. After writing *Is That a Baby. . . .* She delivered her last child, a healthy baby girl, who at the time of publishing, is gleefully tearing up the house. You can contact Anna at *rewight@telusplanet.net.*

T. Brian Kelly is a freelance newspaper and Web editorial cartoonist, humor writer and general wise guy. He is the primary caregiver for his three children, ages four and a half, two and a half and nine months. He is looking forward with great expectation to the end of the diaper years. He lives and works in Oakland, California.

Crystal Kirgiss, a writer and musician, lives in northern Minnesota with her husband, three sons, 120-pound yellow Labrador retriever and seven-pound gray tabby cat.

Elisa Kayser Klein is a media consultant and stay-at-home mom. After her dramatic first pregnancy with Mariel, her dear friend and obstetrician, Dr. Sidney Prescott, went on to help her deliver two more healthy girls, Isabel and Genevieve. An ovarian cancer survivor, Elisa is now chairing a group of cancer support agencies working to build a Cancer Survivors Park in her native Portland, Oregon. Her husband Steven, loves being the father of three little girls.

Susan M. Lang loves learning. It's a good thing, since her two daughters have shown her that parenting is a crash course in discovery. She is a freelance writer and ordained pastor in the ELCA, grateful for the partnership of her husband in their life together.

Jeanne Marie Laskas is a columnist for *The Washington Post Magazine,* where her "Significant Others" essays appear weekly. A contributing writer to *Esquire, Good Housekeeping* and *Health,* she writes for numerous national magazines. She authored *The Balloon Lady and Other People I Know, We Remember,* and her latest book, *Fifty Acres and a Poodle,* a memoir about her life with her husband and daughter, along with their dogs, mules, sheep and other animals on a farm in Pennsylvania.

Claire Simon Lasser is a mother of three and lives with her husband and their children, Catlyne, Chloe and Kyle in Wheaton, Illinois. She owns her own business in Chicago, Illinois, where she is a casting director for television, feature film and commercials.

Audrie LaVigne is a wife, mother, and the assistant director of an agency that works with developmentally disabled adults. She and her husband, Sean, adopted their daughter two years ago from Guatemala. She wrote "To Our Baby Girl" while living in Guatemala with her new daughter, waiting for the adoption to be finalized. She now lives in Northern California with her husband and daughter.

Sharon Linnéa is the producer of the Inspiration Channel at *Beliefnet.com* (where you'll find lots more inspirational stories!). She and her husband, Robert Owens Scott, have two great, though slightly nutty kids, Johnathan and Linnéa. Sharon has enjoyed being a freelance editor for several of the *Chicken Soup for the Soul* books, as well as being a staff writer for *Guideposts* and four other national magazines. Her most recent books are *Princess Kaiulani: Hope of a Nation, Heart of a People;* and *Raoul Wallenberg: The Man Who Stopped Death,* as well as the upcoming *Great American Tree Book* with Jeffrey G. Meyer. Sharon speaks often at writers' conferences as well as to schools on kids' needs for heroes. She can be reached at *Slinnea@warwick.net.*

Barbara Mackey is a professional writer for international corporations as well as national women's magazines such as *Woman's World.* Her favorite topics are women who describe themselves as ordinary but act extraordinarily when challenged by life. Barbara lives in Dayton, Ohio, and Bellaire, Michigan and works worldwide. (Viva la modems!)

Ann Mainse is the daughter of an Army officer and was born in Fort Sam Houston, Texas on September 21, 1963. She lived on various Army bases throughout her childhood and eventually attended Evangel University, in Springfield, Missouri, where she met and married Ron Mainse in July of 1984. Now a full-time stay-at-home mother, Ann volunteers in various Christian ministry-oriented projects, as well as lead a weekly ladies' Bible study. She now resides near Toronto, Canada, with her husband and three children, a daughter and two sons, ages thirteen, ten and seven.

Bonnie J. Mansell lives with her husband and five children in Downey, California, where she teaches memoir-writing classes to help people capture their memories in order to share their stories with their children and grandchildren. She has taught junior high, high school and adult school.

Michelle Mariotti holds a degree in drama from the University of Southern California. She is a devoted wife and the full-time mother of two small sons. Her ultimate dream would be to return to acting, write a screenplay and have her children's stories published. Michelle can be reached at *JNRYSMOM@JUNO.COM.*

Ami McKay lives in Nova Scotia, Canada, with her husband and son. She's a contemporary bard who loves writing, singing and harp playing. Through her arts she hopes to help others recognize their own profound importance in life. To learn more about her current projects, visit: *http://www.hopes.com* or e-mail: *hope@passport.ca.*

Brenda Ford Miller, originally from western New York, now lives in Seminole, Florida. She is first a Christian, married to Jim Miller, and they share six terrific children, four grandchildren and a beloved cat named Abe. Newly retired, they are enjoying traveling among other interests. Brenda enjoys writing and basketry. She is grateful to God for a life full of blessings.

David Mittman is a cofounder of Clinicians Publishing Group, a medical communications company in Clifton, New Jersey. He is a very proud father and, along with his wife, Bonnie, recently celebrated his twenty-fifth wedding anniversary.

Lynn Noelle Mossburg lives in Pittsburgh, Pennsylvania, with her children, Kate, Bethany and Joshua. She feels blessed to teach childbirth education, newborn health, parenting, vaginal birth after cesarean, and hypnobirthing at Allegheny General Hospital, among others. She loves to cuddle babies, read and manage her daughter's band Heartwood. She's greateful for her parents and friends.

Lynne Murphy is a registered nurse from Des Moines, Iowa. She and husband, Morris, are the parents of three children, Taryn, Daniel and Laurel.

Sherrie Page Najarian received her undergraduate degree in nursing from the University of North Carolina and received her master's degree in nursing from Yale University. She is blessed to be married to her amazing, supportive husband, Ed. Currently, Sherrie is a stay-at-home mom raising her two wonderful children, Alexandra and Jonathan.

James A. Nelson is sixty-seven years old with a B.A. in economics from Eastern Washington University. Divorced with seven grandchildren and four children, he has recently self-published a book entitled, *The Way It Was and The Way It Is—Forty-Nine Nostalgic Short Stories.* He has been published many times locally, nationally and internationally.

Mary Ostyn and her husband live in Idaho with their six children, including two Korean-born sons whom they welcomed home in July of 1998 and January 2000. Mary enjoys her days as a full-time mother. Late at night when the house is quiet, she also enjoys writing.

Lynn Plourde is a children's book author. Her picture books include *Pigs in the Mud in the Middle of the Rud, Wild Child,* and *Moose, Of Course!* Lynn lives in Winthrop, Maine, with her husband, two stepsons, and her daughter, Kylee, who was the inspiration for "Seems Like Yesterday."

Ray Recchi was a lifestyle columnist for *The Sun-Sentinel* in Florida. He touched many lives with his humorous and poignant columns about everyday life, many of which were inspired by his own experiences with his wife and children. He is missed by many.

Jennifer Reed has two children, Eric and Emma, a dog, a cat, some goldfish and a hermit crab. Jennifer is stay-at-home mom who enjoys writing, especially for children. She has written for major children's magazines and wishes to publish her children's books.

Carol McAdoo Rehme is a professional storyteller, public speaker, and writer who believes in parenting by the book. Unfortunately, she is still waiting for the right one to be written. Startled to learn that children leave the nest at about the same rate at which they arrived, she watches her own four spreading their wings—before she is ready to let loose. Contact Carol at 2503 Logan Dr., Loveland, CO 80538; phone 970-669-5791 or email her at *crehme@verinet.com.*

Kate Rowinski writes as often as she can, when she is not working at her regular job in the catalog industry. Kate and her husband, Jim, have four children. She has written several books for children as well as for adults. Kate and her family live in Charlottesville, Virginia.

Judy Ryan is a military wife with two beautiful children ages three and six. She has her master's degree in education and considers it a blessing to be called "my teacher." Her favorite word, however is still "mom." She loves to jog, write and spend time with her family.

Elisabeth Sartorius is and always will be "Mom" to her nine children ranging in age from twenty-three to nine years old. Plus, she enjoys being Grams to Elisa's almost two-year-old twins, Sara and Benjamin. Elisabeth is a part-time certified pharmacy technician. In her spare time, she enjoys watching her kids participate in different sports, working in her garden and collecting unusual plants.

Deborah Shouse is a creativity coach, speaker, facilitator and writer. Her work has appeared in *Reader's Digest, Woman's Day* and *Family Circle.* Deborah coauthored *Working Woman's Communications Survival Guide* and *Antiquing for Dummies* (IDG, Spring, 1999). She loves in Prairie Village, Kansas, where she celebrates her anniversary of being a mom.

Robin L. Silverman is the author of *The Ten Gifts*, a pathway to personal peace, and the forthcoming book *Something Wonderful is About to Happen*. Her work also appears in *Chicken Soup for the Unsinkable Soul*, *Heartwarmers* and many national magazines. She lives in Grand Forks, North Dakota with her husband Steve, daughters Amanda and Erica, and their collie, Lady. For more article, book and tape information, see Robin's Web site at *www.robinsilverman.com*.

Joanna Slan is the author of five stories appearing in *Chicken Soup for the Soul* books, making her one of our most popular contributors. *Sharing Ideas* magazine named her one of the top motivational speakers in the world. She is the author of *Scrapbook Storytelling* and *I'm Too Blessed to Be Depressed*. For information, call 1-888-BLESSED.

Nicole Smith is the proud mother of Nicholas, age five, and Elisa, age two. She and her children make their home in Franklin, Indiana. Nicole is currently at work on her first novel and can be reached by email at *sheesh51@hotmail.com*.

Meiji Stewart is the creator of several ABC writings including *Children Need, Loving Families, Great Teachers, Success Is, Friends Are, Dare To*. Many of these are available from Portal Publications at your favorite poster store or directly from *www.hazelden.org* on a variety of gift products. Meiji's PuddleDancer Press is honored to publish Marshall Rosenberg's book *Nonviolent Communication* which Jack Canfield says, "Can literally change the world." Meiji is married to Claudia. He is the father of Malia and stepdad to Tommy. For more information about Meiji's writings or projects, please visit *www.puddledancer.com* or call 858-759-6963.

Cynthia Stewart-Copier (a.k.a. Cindy Barksdale) is a national speaker and the author of several books including *Dream Big! A Woman's Book of Network Marketing* as well as *Dreams of My Own*, and *Keys to Success*, and soon to be released *Creating Wealth on the Web*. Cynthia has been a contributing author to books such as *Chicken Soup for the College Soul, Christmas Miracles* and *The Gift of Miracles*, as well as numerous magazines. She has been on numerous radio and television shows including *The View* with Barbara Walters. Through the many challenges that she has overcome, Cynthia knows first hand how to *dream* big and dedicates her life to empowering other women to stand-up, step-out and reach their dreams. She can be reached at *www.DaretoDreamBig.com*.

Colleen Story is a senior copywriter by profession, but enjoys writing her own stories whenever possible. Her work has appeared in *Country Extra, Nostalgia* and *Once Upon a Time*, among others. She would like to dedicate this poem to her mother, who constantly inspires with her love and encouragement.

Gayle Sorensen Stringer is a mother of three who finds her freelance writing for adults and children cathartic. She holds a master's degree in gifted education and works part time as a gifted facilitator. Holding dear the creative spirit and the mother's heart, she endeavors to use both to touch lives.

Mary Jane Strong has been married for thirty-one years to her husband, David. They have three unusually talented children and one ancient, clever and affectionate but manipulative cat, Patches. She has recently retired from twenty-eight years of teaching, and so has time to spend on her first love, writing. She can be reached at *mjdstrong@hotmail.com* or P.O. Box 383, Woodbury, CT 06789.

Nancy Surella and her husband, Ron, live in Mt. Gilead, Ohio, with their four children. They have adopted both domestically and internationally and remain adoption advocates. Susie has reestablished her relationship with the Surella family. She is now married and the mother of a one-year-old and lives in Germany.

Ken Swarner writes the syndicated humor column, "Family Man," for newspapers in the U.S. and Canada. He lives in the Pacific Northwest with his wife and two children. He can be reached at *noifs@aol.com.*

LeAnn Thieman is a nationally acclaimed speaker and author. A member of the National Speakers Association, LeAnn inspires audiences to balance their lives, truly live their priorities, and make a difference in the world. She has written for seven *Chicken Soup for the Soul* books and is coauthoring *Chicken Soup for the Nurse's Soul.* You can contact LeAnn at 6600 Thompson Drive, Fort Collins, CO 80526; *www.LeAnnThieman.com* or call toll-free 877-THIEMAN.

Jim Warda writes and presents workshops on finding meaning in the moments. He also writes for the Sunday "Family" section of the *Chicago Tribune.* He has a wife, Gina, and two sons, Jeremy and Matthew. Contact 847-642-5108 or subscribe to his free weekly email column at *Wordwind5@aol.com.*

Barbara Warner lives with her husband, Brian and three children outside Dallas, Texas. A former high school English teacher, she is currently an at-home mother and freelance writer. She also has a sister, Laura, who she didn't mention in this story, but loves very much. Her email address is *brian.warner2@gte.net.*

Marion Bond West has written for *Guideposts* for twenty-eight years and is a contributing editor. She has authored six books and is an inspirational speaker. Her first book, *Out of My Bondage,* published in 1976, was subtitled "Required Reading for Every Wife/Mother Who Has Felt Like Screaming." She is the mother of four grown children, including twin sons and she is the grandmother of six. Marion may be reached at 706-353-6523 or by writing to 1330 DaAndra Dr., Watkinsville, Georgia 30677.

Susan Alexander Yates is a bestselling writer and speaker. Her books include *And Then I Had Kids: Encouragement for Mothers of Young Children, What Really Matters at Home: Eight Crucial Elements for Building Character in Your Family* and *How to Like the Ones You Love: Building Family Friendships for Life.* She is the Parent-Child columnist for *Today's Christian Woman* magazine. She and her husband, John, have five children and two grandchildren. They speak at family life conferences throughout the country.

Chicken Soup
for the Whole Family

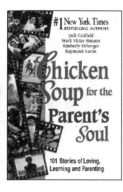

Chicken Soup for the Parent's Soul
Code #7478 • Quality Paperback • $12.95

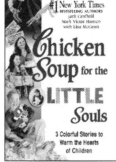

Chicken Soup for Little Souls
Code #8121 • Quality Paperback • $12.95

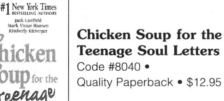

Chicken Soup for the Teenage Soul Letters
Code #8040 •
Quality Paperback • $12.95

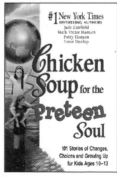

Chicken Soup for the Preteen Soul
Code #8008 • Quality Paperback • $12.95

More Soup to Warm Your Heart

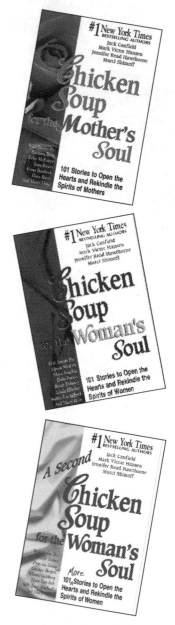

There are many ways to define a woman: daughter, mother, wife, professional, friend, student. . . . We are each special and unique, yet we share a common connection. What bonds all women are our mutual experiences of loving and learning: feeling the tenderness of love; forging lifelong friendships; pursuing a chosen career; giving birth to new life; juggling the responsibilities of job and family, and more.

These three volumes celebrate the myriad facets of a woman's life.

Chicken Soup for the Mother's Soul
Code #4606 Paperback • $12.95

Chicken Soup for the Woman's Soul
Code #4150 Paperback • $12.95

A Second Chicken Soup for the Woman's Soul
Code #6226 Paperback • $12.95

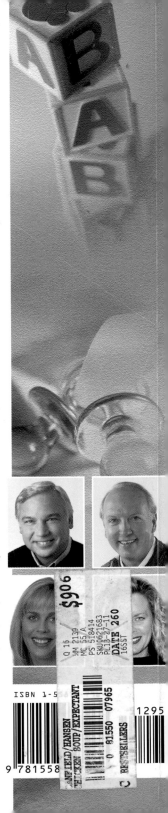

Self-Help/Pregnancy

"Chicken Soup for the Expectant Mother's Soul *captures the anticipation of the most amazing of God's blessings— the miracle of childbirth. This book is inspirational from beginning to end.*"

—**Kathy Ireland**
supermodel and mother

Share the Joy of Expecting a Baby . . .

You watched with anticipation and awe as the test strip turned from white to pink, and thus began the awesome and life-altering adventure of becoming a mother. Whether you're filled with elation, trepidation or a combination of both, *Chicken Soup for the Expectant Mother's Soul* will offer you inspiration as you prepare for the blessed event.

Written by first-time moms, veteran mothers, adoptive mothers and even fathers-to-be, these heartwarming, personal stories share the universal joys and challenges of impending motherhood—from sharing the news with family and friends, to seeing the initial ultrasound, from feeling the first fluttering of life inside you, to finally holding your baby in your arms.

With chapters on Memorable Moments, Small Miracles, Challenges, Expectant Fathers and Special Delivery, this book will tug at your heart, abate any fears, and remind you that, morning sickness and sleep deprivation aside, becoming a mother will bring immeasurable joy and renewed meaning to your life.

Jack Canfield *and* **Mark Victor Hansen,** *the #1* New York Times *and* USA Today *bestselling coauthors of the* Chicken Soup for the Soul *series, have dedicated their lives to the personal and professional development of others.* **Patty Aubery** *is the proud mother of two boys, and the coauthor of* Chicken Soup for the Christian Family Soul, Chicken Soup for the Christian Soul *and* Chicken Soup for the Surviving Soul. **Nancy Mitchell** *is the coauthor of* Chicken Soup for the Christian Family Soul, Chicken Soup for the Christian Soul *and* Chicken Soup for the Surviving Soul.

$12.95

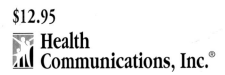

**Health
Communications, Inc.**®

ISBN 1-5

9 781558 0 81550 07965

1295